HEALTH PEACE
AND
THE HOLOGRAPHIC
BODY

The Adventure Begins

MICHAEL A. SCHLEY

BALBOA.
PRESS
A DIVISION OF HAY HOUSE

Balboa Press books may be ordered through booksellers or by contacting:

Balboa Press
A Division of Hay House
1663 Liberty Drive
Bloomington, IN 47403
www.balboapress.com
1 (877) 407-4847

Because of the dynamic nature of the Internet, any web addresses or links contained in this book may have changed since publication and may no longer be valid. The views expressed in this work are solely those of the author and do not necessarily reflect the views of the publisher, and the publisher hereby disclaims any responsibility for them.

The author of this book does not dispense medical advice or prescribe the use of any technique as a form of treatment for physical, emotional, or medical problems without the advice of a physician, either directly or indirectly. The intent of the author is only to offer information of a general nature to help you in your quest for emotional and spiritual well-being. In the event you use any of the information in this book for yourself, which is your constitutional right, the author and the publisher assume no responsibility for your actions.

Any people depicted in stock imagery provided by Thinkstock are models, and such images are being used for illustrative purposes only.
Certain stock imagery © Thinkstock.

Print information available on the last page.

ISBN: 978-1-5043-6687-8 (sc)
ISBN: 978-1-5043-6688-5 (hc)
ISBN: 978-1-5043-6689-2 (e)

Library of Congress Control Number: 2016915690

Balboa Press rev. date: 10/24/2016

Beyond our own personal choice and responsibility for our life and its context, which is definitive, everyone has many people to whom they owe their life experiences, education, and feeling of self-worth, being loved, cared about, and cared for. It is to these people and you readers I dedicate this book.

Here are some of the people who have contributed to me.

For my wife, Vicki, who is also an author and who lovingly dedicated herself to the task of the first edit of this book. I love you forever. You are the person in this world I have the most fun with.

To Connie, who loved me and taught me a lot, and with whom I spent many great years raising Pancho and Carol. I loved you, and you left us too soon.

For my children, Carol, Pancho, Gabrielle, Aaron, Veronica, and Bret, and their remarkable children. I will always love you. Thank you for being you.

For my granddaughter, Mattie, who is an aspiring writer and who helped me choose the title of this book. I will always love you. Thank you for being you.

For my mother, who, above all, gave me the experience of a mother's love and commitment, the blessed holoprinter, without whom I would have had no physical existence in this apparently three-dimensional world, and second, my father who participated at a soul level in my creation, who loved my mother and me, and whom my mother loved more than any other husband during her life.

For my first stepfather, Carlos, who told me about a priest who could heal people by looking in their eyes and taught me how to play chess, how to repair almost anything mechanical, and how to speak Spanish well enough to get along. He gave me my first set of mechanical drawing tools and showed me how to draw my first complex compass image, which I came to recognize as the "Seed of Life," an ancient universal key to our holographic universe and our holographic body. For my second stepfather, Jimmy, who, after asking for my permission, dedicated his life to my mother and me and taught me that unconditional love and caring is the most important thing in the world. For my brother, Richard, who one summer taught me the trade of landscaping and gardening, as well as math as it relates to owning your own business.

For Dr. Bernard Jensen, naturopath, chiropractor, and iridologist, who I consider to be the father of modern American iridology and who taught me about natural health, healing, and iridology (the science of reading the iris of the eye, which shows the relative balance of the entire body). He was as excited as I was about the subject of color and healing and shared with me his extensive collection of color healing devices.

For Cindy, the teacher of my first Touch for Health class. For Dr. John Thie, Dr. Mary Marks, Seth, and Grace, without whom the first *Touch for Health* book, and the "Touch for Health" natural health, acupuncture touch, and massage approach to restoring our natural energies may have never existed and become popular worldwide, continuing to benefit millions of people around the world. For Gordon Stokes and Shanti Moore, early trainers for "Touch for Health" instructors, of which I was one. Thank you. For Dr. John Thie, who asked me if I would and then gave me the privilege of helping to organize and be chairman of the first (1981) and then the second (1982) International Touch for Health Worldwide conferences in San Diego, California.

For Dr. Carey Reams, who I had the good fortune to meet and do a workshop with, getting exposed to the Reams biological theory of ionization. By using urine and saliva testing, Dr. Reams has given people foolproof information on how they can maintain and balance their body, which will then heal itself of almost any imbalance.

For Dr. Marcel Vogel (holder of a great number of patents for liquid crystalline and bioluminescent devices), who shared with me his experience of witnessing the flash of blue light that occurs at the point of human conception and who was a living example of someone who had a comprehensive grasp of our energetic relationship to each other and our universe.

For James W. Dilley, bookstore owner who mentored a once angry young man, teaching him to leave space for those who seem to disagree with you and showing him how, with intention, attention, and caring, not only is the impossible possible, but the realization almost always exceeds the imagining.

For the great spiritual leaders of all true faiths, who we can recognize by their teaching the need to care for and love each other, that we are all part of a greater spiritual family, teaching compassion and inclusion, that there is no separation.

For Dinshah P. Ghadiali, author of the three-volume *Spectrochrometry Encyclopedia*, the "Parsee Edison" scientist, vegan, and color, health, and healing advocate and practitioner, whose work informed mine and who, in spite of being persecuted and jailed for his original work, which was and still is definitive in the field of color in relation to health, never denied the truths he knew would eventually prevail.

For Darius Dinshah, author of *Let There Be Light*, son of Dinshah, who years ago kindly met with me and shared additional information about his father's work and the Dinshah Health Society.

And last but not least, for all of you who want to, have, or are now contributing to our world by living a path of true peace and light, living a life of looking out for one another, I thank you and offer these words: "We all travel, with each other, each as sister, each as brother. Is it any wonder that I call you friend?"

CONTENTS

FOREWORD

Michael Schley is a gentleman with a gentle soul; a
philosopher and an activist; and a practitioner of and
advocate for peace, health, and fulfillment.
In this book, he offers practical suggestions and encouragement
for living a healthful, peaceful, happy life. I acknowledge and
thank Michael for sharing this knowledge and recommend
that you read the book and use it as a guide on your
journey of life. There is great wisdom in his words.
Namaste,
Cliff Popejoy, author of *Stanley Easy Home Wiring Repairs*

PREFACE

I invite you to join me in the pages of this book to participate in possibly the greatest adventure of your life! Of course you will have to pay very close attention, or you will miss it! Sometimes the treasure is in the ground, and sometimes it is in an old chest hidden away in the back of an attic, or a cave, or a hidden storeroom. And sometimes the treasure is in plain sight, and because we have not learned to look with new eyes, we miss it! This book came into being because I wanted you, the reader, to have in one book some of the very best and most valuable information that has been shared with me and that I have discovered in my lifelong study of health and healing, as well as from my thirty-seven years (so far) as a health consultant, certified massage therapist, life coach, applied kinesiology practitioner, and holographic body worker. This book is a practical, prioritized guide to health, happiness, and discovery. If you adopt this book as a lifelong friend, you will come to understand why I say it is a definition and an experience that explains and identifies the nature or essential qualities of life! The context and content of this book is in the title's definitions.
Health is derived from hale or whole, as in whole in body, mind, and spirit, balanced, centered, feeling vigorous, vital, and at ease.
Peace is experiencing health (as noted above), a
normal state of individual and mutual harmony,
people or groups getting along with each other.

Holographic body refers to our physical body and the whole (holy) body. Like a holographic photo negative, where the smallest piece of the negative portrays the entire picture, with the physical body and the whole (holy) body, the smallest piece also portrays the entire body; we only need to know how to read and experience this. This book will give you tools to access your holographic body and database, the gateway to discovery.

The point is there is only now. After a moment ago is now. The experience, now, is an introduction to now. What is now? When we know now, backwards and forwards, we have won the present.

INTRODUCTION

I invite you to look at this book with new eyes, as if you were just beginning to really live. Pretend that you have just entered a miraculous time, and you are expanding your sense ability! Like the first time you breathed, drank water, tasted food, moved your body, saw colors, or were aware of your heart and mind. Everything is bright, new, and exciting, a miraculous world of unlimited possibility.

My mother and father were very much in love at the time, doing what people do just prior to my conception. There was a flash of blue light—and eureka! The *holoprint* of my existence was transferred to what we call the human genetic material of our three-dimensional world. Holoprint is a word I have invented to cover the concept of the photocopying transfer of information from the universal holographic field, in this particular case, through the sperm/ovum heart-connected impregnation of my mother. Having found a receptive and fully functional, switched-on *holographic copy* producer, the new holoprint, through the gracious cooperation of my mother, spent the next nine months holoprinting my apparently three-dimensional existence into the physical. The term *holoprinting* provides you a model of light-transferred information capable of providing the apparently three-dimensional blueprint of a live, breathing human being. We have an opportunity from the time we are born to the time we die to learn exciting new things and to participate in a great adventure.

CHAPTER 1

Breathing

Number one in importance—make sure you keep
breathing available, pure, toxin-free, clean air. It is good
if you can put yourself in the healthiest air possible.
This can be accomplished in a number of ways—some
of which I will list here for your consideration.
Get an air washing and purification system for your home or a
portable unit for the room you spend the most time in (if you live in
a toxic-air area and moving does not seem feasible). The investment
will more than repay itself in your added health. Finding a
healthy-air environment and moving there is another possibility.
If the above suggestions seem too difficult or not currently
possible, then consider at least conditioning the air in your
home with an inexpensive ion generator (or two). Run them in
the rooms in your home where you spend the most time. The
older used ones can often be found in thrift or secondhand
stores for a few dollars. They work fine for settling dust out
of the air, and though you may have to dust more often, at
least you won't be breathing it! Don't run these all the time,
just until you see a good amount of dust settled on surfaces,
or after dusting or running a vacuum, or on dusty days.
Get a good-quality spray bottle and occasionally mist the air
in your home. I use one of the following solutions for misting:
plain pure water, distilled water, or water to which I have added

hydrogen peroxide in a ratio of one tablespoon to half a gallon of water. This will wash the air and add negative ions to the air (useful for healing and a sense of well-being). Water with hydrogen peroxide also adds oxygen to the air. Make sure not to use this misting in an already humid environment or in spaces where you are not going to be. A good rule of thumb would be once a day, to a maximum of three or four times per day if you are in a dry environment. In extremely dry environments or if using wood for winter heating, up to five or six times per day could be possible.

Breathing exercises can also be very important to our health. It is reasonable to say that breath is life!

Here is the Schley Conscious Breathing Training Technique. Pay conscious attention to your breathing at least three times per day and check the following: are you a relaxed breather or a tense breather? Relaxed breathers tend to allow the relaxed body to take in the air and distribute it as required. Tense breathers tend to tense certain muscle sets and related body areas each time they breathe, which can lead to various physical complaints and real body concerns, such as tight neck and shoulders, tight chest, tension-induced circulation issues, pain, and a host of other concerns. It is to your advantage to identify what type of breather you are and then retrain yourself to breathe for optimal health.

If you are a tense breather, your first action is to learn how to be a relaxed breather. Take the Schley Conscious Breathing Training Techniques as described below and apply them to any tense, uncomfortable, or out-of-balance areas of the body you are aware of, until you become a relaxed breather.

If you are a relaxed breather, you have a certain advantage in that you do not have to do much to train yourself to relax. There are not a lot of people who are completely relaxed breathers, so you may wish to include tune-ups during your three conscious periods of breathing each day.

Consciously direct your breath to areas where you want to release tension, heal, improve vitality, increase circulation, and expand your awareness. This process of directed breathing can be achieved by imagining your whole body is breathing in and out, even your skin. Breathe in a full breath, imagining that this breath is going to certain directed areas of your body, and imagine that you are experiencing the desired effect of this breath, such as healing, relaxation, improved circulation, improved vitality, eliminated discomfort, and generally improved health. Now breathe out wholly and completely, simply reversing the breathing-in process, even breathing out through your skin, allowing the outgoing breath to eliminate any toxins and respiratory waste materials. We call this breath a "round breath," in that the breath is not held at any point. It is as though the breath is drawing a circle, with the *in* breath being the first half of the circle and the *out* breath being the second half of the circle. Most people, by consciously focusing on and experiencing different parts of the body, can identify and balance any tense, uncomfortable, and out-of-balance areas using the Schley conscious breathing training, directed breathing, and relaxation techniques. It is possible that you can be unaware of areas of tension or imbalance and that even after you have consciously focused on different body areas, some tense or blocked areas may still not be discovered. You can be assisted in discovering these areas by enlisting the help of caring friends or natural health care professionals, particularly therapeutic massage and breath therapists, physical therapists, chiropractors, yoga teachers, tai chi or chi gong instructors, and kinesiology health professionals who are aware of whole body dynamics in relation to health. We have now covered simple breathing basics. As in all the important subjects of this book, one could spend an entire lifetime studying breathing and would find that the study and practice of breathing alone will ultimately provide a holographic map to body balance, super consciousness, and relationships to the holographic body generally unknown to the public at large.

For those of you who have found this subject exceptionally interesting, I refer you to the bibliography (references and resources by chapter) at the end of this book for more information.

3

CHAPTER 2

Water

Do not underestimate the value of pure water in the maintenance of your health. Since the majority of our bodies consist of water, it is only reasonable that we make the purity, quality, and amount of water we put into our bodies a priority project! Water is also life! To begin with, research and find out about the quality of the water you have been drinking on a regular basis. You may have to pay for an independent analysis to get truly accurate information. If your water is pure and of good quality, great! If not, check on the availability of pure water in your area. If you find a reasonable, trusted source of pure water (which may not be as easy as it sounds), then your drinking water problem is solved. I recommend drinking a full glass of distilled water (or two if you are thirsty) first thing in the morning, before drinking or eating anything else. If possible, give your body twenty minutes or more to assimilate this new water. The average adult can use eight to twelve eight-ounce glasses of water per day, or more depending on the amount of physical activity the person does. When you are thirsty, that is your body letting you know you need water. Drink pure water and stay adequately hydrated. Distilled water purchased from the store is much better than most tap water; however, occasionally too much plastic transfers from the plastic bottle to the water. This most often happens during the summer, when the water being transported gets overheated in the

4

plastic. If you can find distilled water in glass bottles, that is ideal. Most tap water is like a passenger train with all or most of the seats on the train occupied and little or no space for passengers. Distilled water is like the same train with all or most of the seats on the train available for passengers. When you drink distilled water first thing in the morning, the passengers on this distilled water train are the waste materials your body has been producing during your sleep, and since the train has arrived, your body will make sure as many of these waste materials as possible take the train out of the body. In addition, any material the body needs to transfer to some other location can take a short hop on this train and get off at the location needed before the distilled water train leaves the body. Pure water, as noted earlier, is a transport facilitator and medium for nutrients and minerals to be more easily dispersed where needed in the body, as well as transporting waste materials out of the body. Energy can be imprinted into water, and that energy can be transferred to someone using this water for washing or drinking. This subject alone could be, and has been, the subject of a number of books. I believe, and it has been recorded, that the power of prayer and intention can and does alter the energetic structure of water. Since we are mostly water, what can the power of prayer and intention do for us? We will refer to this idea again in the section on the *holographic body*. There are people, and I happen to be one of them, who believe "new water" is being continually created deep in the earth and that this water finds its way to the surface in select geological areas. If you are aware of these areas, or if you happen to own one of these new water wells or springs, consider that you have one of the most valuable resources of the world in your possession! If you know of someone who owns or knows the location of one or more of these new water wells, consider purchasing water rights to a percentage of this pure water. If you have friends who own one of these new water wells or springs and they are willing to share with you, consider that you have been gifted with a treasured resource through their kindness. There are

5

also wells and aquifers that are still producing pure and clean water, although they are becoming harder to find. If you find or own one of these, celebrate. If you have an interest in pure water—and we all should—just discovering and identifying these water sources and making agreements with the owners or purchasing the sources could be a valuable undertaking.

If you do not have access to pure water, you must do the best you can. Most supermarkets and healthy food stores carry distilled water. They also often carry inexpensive bulk drinking water that is double reverse osmosis, carbon filtered, ultraviolet light-treated purified water that you can fill your own container with, or purchase a container to fill. I personally have used water filtration, double reverse osmosis water purification systems, and portable home kitchen water distillers. If finding pure or distilled water is too much trouble and you have a reliable electrical source, I would recommend you consider buying a portable kitchen water distiller. Whatever you choose to do, please start your day, before eating anything, by drinking at least one or two glasses (if you are thirsty) of distilled water. If you have a good solar location, you could also experiment with a solar distiller; either buy or build one. As in all primary categories in this book, water can also be a fulfilling lifetime study. See the bibliography (reference and resources by chapter) at the end of this book for more information.

CHAPTER 3

Food

Be a Rainbow Eater (people like you, committed to living a healthy life, in a peaceful world, where win/win solutions are a way of life!) Rainbow Eaters select vegetables and fruits including all the colors of the rainbow which provide, not only colorful food, but a full spectrum of nutrition. When possible, eat organically grown food. It is better if you can find your food locally grown. Properly grown, organically certified food is generally higher in vital energy and true, useable nutritional value, including enzymes, trace elements, and minerals. Avoid commercially, chemically grown, pesticide-sprayed, possibly GMO-altered, irradiated food (GMO stands for genetically modified organism, more commonly referred to as genetically modified foods). Sometimes organically grown and certified food is a bit more expensive than commercially grown food; however, your body will know the difference. You and your family will not have to deal with the impact and elimination of the toxic material that is often inside or on the surface of commercially grown, toxic, chemical food. Here are two valuable shopping tips that you can train yourself to notice. When shopping for food, select the item that you are considering buying by looking at it before you touch it. Notice while standing still if your body is making a micro-movement toward the item (leaning toward it) or away from the item (leaning away from it). This movement is sometimes quite obvious and sometimes very subtle, but, anyone with a little practice can train themselves to notice this. Initially, get a friend to observe you, as it is sometimes easier for a separate party to notice the movements in the beginning. Just have your friend notice, while you are standing still, if you lean toward or away from the item being considered. If your body leans toward the item, that is an indicator that it is probably good for you; if your body leans away from the item, it is probably not good for you. Our holographic sensory systems, which have developed over the centuries, have trained our holographic body to notice this as a matter of survival. When we have trained ourselves in these practices, we can train others. If you are a visually oriented person, you can train yourself to notice another indicator, which is the color of live food, such as fruits and vegetables. Food that is not healthy for human consumption has a "shadow field" on and around it. Train yourself to see this field by relaxing and viewing your intended purchase with "soft eyes," consciously relaxing your gaze and noticing an almost floating, shadowy gray mist on and around the item or items. Buy those without shadows. Avoid those with shadows. One of the easiest foods to train on is apples, as they are quite easy to see the difference on. Do not be surprised to find that many or most items have shadows, even in health-food stores! These two shopping tips are simple, easy examples. Processed foods are not live foods but do have a discernible energy field. I do not believe that there is a way for you to be fooled into buying something unhealthy for you once you have learned these two practices! There are many methods we can use to train ourselves to know what is good for us. Another practice is to use muscle testing when selecting foods. General guidelines for muscle testing can be found in chapter 9. Training yourself is the best investment you can make for your health and the health of those you love! Once you are trained, you will know without a doubt what is good for you and not good for you. Be a Rainbow Eater.

Start with Red Foods. Eat Your Beets.

Grate raw red beets. The grating process exposes the vegetable to the air and changes it from a kind of bitter vegetable to a mildly sweet and delicious vegetable that your body will love! Said to build the blood, beets are high in available nutrients that nourish the blood.

Orange Foods. Eat Your Carrots.

Here again, grated raw carrots are delicious and a great source of calcium and carotene for the body. Ever see that white stuff in the bottom of a bottle of carrot juice? That's calcium! I recommend carrots. There are many different orange foods to choose from, including raw and grated butternut squash or pumpkin for example.

Yellow Foods. Eat Your Squash.

Crookneck squash, raw and grated, is a good yellow food. An additional good yellow food is spaghetti squash, a delightful vegetable alternative to the pasta in spaghetti. Juice of a ripe yellow, organically grown Meyer lemon, or any other lemon, makes great lemonade, just plain in distilled water (good first thing in the morning). If too tart, add a small amount of organic, pure maple syrup to taste. And of course this lemon juice with a little cold pressed olive oil and some herbs and seasonings makes a good, healthy salad dressing. Again, there are many different yellow foods to choose from.

Green Foods. Eat your greens.

Green food, food high in chlorophyll, has a cleansing and blood-nourishing effect on the body. The chlorophyll molecule is very similar to the hemoglobin molecule of the blood. Green is one of the primary balancing colors of the body. Green foods, such as sprouts of all kinds (I love sunflower seed sprouts), are good green food and full of life! Wheat grass is also good; just chew the grass or drink the juice. Some people do not care for wheat grass, but it has a long track record for being extremely healthy.

If you choose to grow your own wheat grass in flats of soil, be sure to add some kelp meal to the soil. Kelp meal increases the vitality of the wheatgrass, adding important trace minerals and nutrients. If you do not care for wheat grass (or have a wheat grass sensitivity), growing sprouts of other vegetables is a good alternative. Consider growing your own sprouts in your kitchen (from organically certified non-GMO seeds). It's easy!

There are so many good greens out there, such as broccoli, Brussel sprouts, green beans, cabbage, kale, mustard greens, and an almost endless variety of other edible greens. You won't have any problem finding green foods! While it is always more desirable to eat our vegetables in their raw state as fresh as possible, the practice of juicing for adding vegetables and fruits to our bodies when we need it is helpful when we have not been able to consume enough vegetables and fruits. One of my favorite vegetable and fruit drink combinations is carrot, kale (or spinach), celery, red beets, and apple juice. Very yummy! You will have to play with the amounts of each until you determine what is perfect at any given time for you.

Blue Foods. Eat Your Blueberries.

Blueberries are a good blue food. Another good one is flax seed oil and flax seed, which is also very good for you. Take my word for it—this is a blue food! Ever see a flax seed plant flower? Bright blue!

Indigo/Violet Foods. Eat your Berries.

Blackberries, blue corn, and some grapes are indigo/
violet foods. Violet foods also include purple cabbage,
eggplant, and the flower of the violet plant.

These suggestions are not exclusive, so be sure to select
your own favorite vegetables in a variety of colors for your
continuing adventure in the Rainbow Eaters Group. There
you have some basic rainbow eaters' instructions.
When you adopt the recommendations in this book, one of the
things that will happen is that your body will begin to develop
an alkaline reserve, which is an optimally functioning healthy
body. The acid/alkaline balance of your body is a good indicator
of whether or not you are successfully maintaining a healthy
body. You can do home pH testing by purchasing Litmus paper
from almost any drugstore or health-food store and test your own
saliva and/or urine. The ideal range for saliva and urine is 6.0 to
6.8. If we maintain a constant average pH 6.4 for saliva and 6.4
for urine, we will probably consider ourselves in good health.
The tests should be done in the morning before eating or at
least an hour after eating. If you set up a consistent testing
system (same times, three times per day, for example), you will
have more ability to adjust your lifestyle to balance your pH.
The testing paper will change color to indicate whether your
system is more alkaline or acid. You quickly dip enough of the
paper in the saliva or urine to lightly wet it and then compare
the color to the color chart that indicates the pH numbers.
If you find you are too acidic, reduce or eliminate the acid-forming
foods, liquids, and behaviors until you return to the ideal average
saliva and urine pH 6.4. An example of one acid-forming food is
red meat. One acid-forming liquid would be carbonated sugary
soft drinks. One acid-creating behavior is stress. You may also
add more alkaline foods, liquids, and behaviors to your routine.
An example of one alkaline food is the king of alkalizers, the

umeboshi plum. You can find it in most health and natural food stores. One alkalizing liquid is lemon juice and distilled water; even though the lemon is citric acid, it creates an alkaline reaction in the body. One example of an alkalizing behavior is quietly being present to whatever gives you the feeling of thankfulness or gratitude. If your tests show you to be too alkaline, then reduce the alkalizers and increase the acid-forming foods.

Try this experiment. Get a blood test from a natural health company that shows a full panel and profile of blood health and explains the tests. Then for thirty days, eat a rainbow! Eat whatever you usually do; only include a full spectrum of vegetables (the ones we describe here are ideal). Make sure you include at least three different color vegetable servings every day (that is twenty-one servings of vegetables each week). The servings do not have to be large. Then return for another blood test with the same panel and profile and compare the two. You may be pleasantly surprised!

I love life, I love color, I love food, and I love eating and experiencing the energy of organic, natural, fresh, live foods in all their variations—whole, fresh, sliced, chopped, julienned, sculpted, ground, grated, dried, pickled, toasted, brewed, and roasted! I love different tastes, looks, smells, sensations, sounds, and everything about the delicious experiences of eating and sharing food. I love sharing life experiences with loved ones. So I have to share this next fun section!

Chocolate, Olive Oil, Coffee, and Tea

Many people live their whole lives engaged in and passionate about something to do with chocolate, olive oil, coffee, and tea. Everything can be better with chocolate, olive oil, coffee, and tea. I mean not just any chocolate, olive oil, coffee, and tea. I mean great chocolate, olive oil, coffee, and tea! Fortunately, there is and has been a long history of people committed to responsibly selecting, wild harvesting, growing, and creating the best chocolate, olive oil, coffee, and tea in the world. Like anything else, when we are consciously striving for great quality, purity, and taste, everything associated with our subject becomes important. Everything—including where each item is grown, the selection of what is grown, the climate, soil type, growing methods, water, and seasons—is taken into consideration. After growing comes harvesting and how we handle, store, and share these crops in the most responsible, efficient, and quality-conscious way. Every human being who is engaged in, loves, and is passionate about what they are doing is usually having fun! When we are having fun, everything becomes a source of inspiration, marvel, and magic. The life experiences and processes that chocolate, olive oil, coffee, and tea plants go through play a role in determining the quality and refinement, flavor, and impact of the finished products. Our life experiences and processes that we as human beings go through also play a determining role in our life and its quality refinement, flavor and impact. The difference between us and fine chocolate, olive oil, coffee, and tea is that their life experiences and processes for the most part are a result of what has been done to them. While it can be said that we as human beings may have been impacted by what has been done to us, our life experiences and processes are determined by the choices we have made either consciously, or unconsciously, and our life and the quality of our life, its flavor, and impact are a direct result of those choices. Fine chocolate, olive oil, coffee, and tea do not get to choose each and every moment of their lives how their life is going to go; we, on the other hand, get to choose each and every moment of our lives how our life is going to go! Whether we make these choices or even know that these choices are available to us is a matter of our consciousness. When we are responsibly committed to growing and creating a great life for ourselves, everything associated with our subject (our life) becomes important.

If you want to love life, love color, love food, love sharing life experiences with loved ones, love the different tastes, looks, smells, sensations, sounds, and delicious variations and experiences of life, and if you want to have a life with wonderful quality, content, and context, begin by having fun and paying attention to everything, because everything associated with our subject is important! Get some friends together for a great tasting experience! This is a time when you can choose what to taste, using chocolate, as an example—four to six chocolates of different origins (say Africa, France, Mexico, and South America) is a good number. A nice event is to taste, share your experiences about the tastings, and then get informed about what was tasted. I suggest that after the tastings you take time to share with each other what your experiences were, the tastes, feelings, smells, and the differences in the different samples. Whether it is chocolate, olive oil, coffee, or tea, use your imagination. I also love street food! I suggest that while you are sharing, if you really enjoy the experience with your friends, also share with them what you are thankful about or appreciate about their friendship and your shared experiences.

Then allow your life to be as great as you can imagine it.

See the bibliography at the end of this book for additional information. As in previous chapters, you could spend a lifetime studying or doing projects indicated by any one of these categories, and with a consciousness of contributing, you would contribute immensely to yourself, your family, your society, and our world!

CHAPTER 4

Herbivore, Omnivore, Carnivore?

Who are you? Are you an herbivore, a person who eats vegetables and fruits? Are you an omnivore, a person who eats vegetables, fruits, and a selection of various eggs, milk, and meats? Are you a carnivore, a person who eats just meat and no fruits and vegetables? Generally speaking, the colder the climate you live in, the more likely you are to be a carnivore. As we move to the more temperate areas, or tropical climates, the more likely we are to be an omnivore or herbivore. There are, however, in all climate zones humans and animals in each of these three categories. There are herbivores in the Arctic, in temperate zones, and in the tropics, and there are omnivores and carnivores in these areas also. So what is the purpose of this chapter? The purpose of this chapter is to allow us to take a look at how we eat and to determine if it may be to our advantage to consider other ways of eating. For example, there are many eating variations and cultural preferences (based on what was available where people lived), and they often include belief structures related to those cultures. There are also those who choose to be vegetarian or vegan. A vegetarian does not eat meat, fish, or poultry, and a vegan does not eat any food derived from animals, which includes eggs, milk, and cheese. It is well known that vegetarians generally live ten to twenty-five years longer and have less illness and disease.

Do we want to consider becoming vegetarian or vegan? It has

also been suggested that your blood type may offer information for the best food choices for you to include in your diet. Something else to consider is this: are you willing to kill the chicken, turkey, cow, pig, lamb, or goat, and butcher it, cut it up, and grind the meat for your dinner? If not, have you given any thought to how your dinner selections are being killed and prepared? Do you think that those processes contribute to the feeling of peace in the world or to the feeling of terror and pain? If you are willing to kill your dinner and eat meat, then perhaps you can consider continuing to eat how you are now; if not, then perhaps you could consider changing your diet. If you choose to eat beef, it should be grass fed. All meat should be naturally grown, organically fed, certified with no antibiotics, GMO, or hormones. Chickens should be free range, naturally grown, and organically fed (no antibiotics, GMO, or hormones), as well as eggs that you purchase. Fish should be wild caught. Do not eat fish that is an introduced species or a farmed species grown with antibiotics, chemicals, and colorings. If you have meat, chicken, or fish on your eating list, consider that the volume consumed is important. As a guideline, meat or fish of any kind should not be more than one-seventh of anyone's diet. For each pound of food consumed, meat or fish should not exceed two to three ounces. The bulk of our eating should consist of organically grown vegetables and fruits with sprouts, grains, and beans added as needed.

If we are basically peaceful people, then perhaps it makes sense to eat more peaceful food. Is a food less peaceful if you or someone else had to kill it and butcher it? Probably. Many people in the world adopt and practice the idea of "Ahimsa" (do no harm). This applies to all of life, including what we eat. If we adopt the idea of "do no harm," then we are making the world a safer/healthier place for us and everyone else, whether we see it or not. We are what we eat, what we think, who we are being, and most of all how we connect with each other at the heart level. Take a look at how you are eating, thinking, and connecting with the world around you and see if you wish to choose a different style or not. I am currently an omnivore, meaning I eat meat, dairy, eggs, vegetables, and fruits. I do not eat anything I would not be willing to kill. On its face, this means I am not as peaceful or balanced as I could be. I have been a vegan in the past and was healthy and energetic. There is no question in my mind or heart that the "do no harm" lifestyle is a preferred way to live. If we eat only that which is freely offered to us, such as fruits, grains, seeds, and vegetables, then we are in effect doing no harm. Personally, I am moving once again in the direction of do no harm. Let us take a look at how we are eating, thinking, feeling, and connecting at the heart level. Now choose what we already have, or perhaps something else that we might prefer.

For additional information, see the bibliography at the end of this book.

CHAPTER 5

Exercise

Getting at least forty-five minutes of aerobic exercise three times per week and walking a minimum distance of two miles at least three times per week, in addition to your regular activity, is a good idea and represents a good program for staying in shape. You can do ten to twelve four-minute aerobic sessions over the course of the day if you feel you cannot do forty-five minutes all at once. The four-minute workout is divided into twenty seconds of aerobic work and a ten-second break; repeat until you total four minutes. If you are not in shape and have not been exercising, you may have to start by doing considerably less and working up to the four minutes by doing twenty seconds of aerobics and resting until you can do another twenty seconds. Congratulate yourself for what you are doing! Do not put yourself down for what you are not doing! Remember, in most cases, it is that much more than you were doing! Gradually, easily, allow yourself to increase your aerobic exercise times until you increase your exercise regimen to the recommended forty-five minutes three times per week in addition to walking two miles (minimum) three times per week. You do not need any equipment to do these exercises. You can start by doing a variety of exercises just using your own body weight. The important thing is to start now! Do what you can right now! Start walking and note the distance you can walk. Stop when you tire and then go again when you are rested. You will find that each day you

can do a little more and are a bit more capable than the day before.
Do your aerobic exercise in the same way, allowing yourself to gradually increase your aerobic times without overdoing it. Start with some modified push-ups (knees-down push-ups) where you are not lifting your full body weight. Every time you do push-ups, do a few more until you graduate to full push-ups and beyond! Do the same with sitting knee bends, then standing knee bends, then knee bends supporting your body weight (squats), developing a program for yourself that includes exercises for your whole body. A helpful hint is that the exercises we least like are probably the exercises we need the most. Sit-ups or abdominal work often falls into this category. Every exercise you do that contracts muscles, such as lifting weights, pull-ups, or supporting your body doing push-ups, should be balanced with an equal amount of time stretching and relaxing. Let's say during a one-week period you walk two miles three times (a total of six miles) in addition to your regular walking. Ideally you would walk two miles one day and do a forty-five-minute aerobic exercise workout, including focusing on the part of your body that needs the most attention. The next day, play, relax, allow, extend, twist, rotate, stretch, bend, and do full range of motion, muscle movements. Practice your Schley Conscious Breathing Training (see chapter 1) tuning into your "being" body as you practice directed breathing and relaxation techniques. The next day, repeat day one. Walk two miles minimum (or whatever you have allowed yourself to work up to) and do forty-five minutes of aerobic exercise (or whatever you have allowed yourself to work up to). The next day, repeat day two: play, relax, allow, extend, twist, rotate, stretch, and bend, tuning into your "being" body as you practice directed breathing and relaxation techniques. Your workout routine would begin to look like this:

- **Monday**—Go walk two miles (or whatever you can do, gradually increasing until you are able to walk at least two miles) and do whatever amount of aerobic exercise you can, allowing yourself gently (don't overdo) to work up to a total of forty-five minutes.

- **Tuesday**—play, relax, allow, extend, twist, rotate, stretch, and bend, incorporating gentle, full-range-of-motion movements for the entire body. Tune into you're "being" body as you do the above, and practice your directed breathing and relaxation techniques.
- **Wednesday**—Walk two miles (or whatever you can do, gradually increasing until you are able to walk at least two miles) and do whatever amount of aerobic exercise you can, allowing yourself gently (don't overdo) to work up to a total of forty-five minutes.
- **Thursday**—Play, relax, allow, extend, twist, rotate, stretch, and bend all muscles while practicing *being* and doing directed breathing and relaxation techniques.
- **Friday**—Walk two miles (or whatever you have worked up to). Then do forty-five-minute aerobic workout (or whatever you have worked up to). Don't forget to work on body muscle areas that need more development.
- **Saturday**—Play, relax, allow, extend, stretch, rotate, twist, and bend all muscles of the body while *being* and doing directed breathing, and relaxation techniques.
- **Sunday**—Rest, relax, play, imagine, create, and pray.

Definitions

Rest and relax—refreshing quiet, repose of sleep, mental or spiritual calm, refreshing ease, or inactivity after exertion or labor, relief of tension, loosening, freedom, solitude, tranquility.

Play—freedom of action, or scope of activity.

Imagine—to form a mental image, create, or invent with the mind.

Create—to cause to come into being, something from your own thought or imagination.

Pray—to give thanks, to ask ("Ask and ye shall receive").

Take Sunday to relax, heal, and breathe as noted earlier in book. Take this day to get in touch with your body and sense what areas seem to be strong and what areas seem to be less strong. Incorporate into your workout routine the following weekly exercises that will strengthen those areas you feel are not as strong, giving them a chance to strengthen as well. Remember, the recommended routine is to walk and do aerobic workout one day, then the next day relax and stretch those muscles you worked out the previous day. Note that at the end of one week, you are considerably more capable than you were the week before. Don't stop. Continue walking, extending your distance as you are able, and increasing your workout routines, adding refinements as you go. When you continue this routine every week, you will notice you are more capable, flexible, energetic, and vital.

The ideal would be to exercise all the muscles of the body through their complete range of motion regularly. Then the next day relax and stretch your muscles so that you wind up with a strong, flexible, well-shaped body that anyone would be glad to have! Make this a lifestyle and you will find yourself in shape, feeling vital, youthful, and alive. When you have exercised for fourteen to thirty days, you will begin to notice that some muscle groups are not as strong as others.

Consider that every muscle in the body should be at maximum strength and flexibility in proportion to its size and the job it needs to do. Naturally the triceps will not be as strong as the quadriceps because they are different sizes and have different functions, but we want all muscles to be in optimal shape and condition for their form and function. You will begin to notice that muscles work in complementary sets and that full extension and contraction of one set of muscles also has full extension and contraction of the complementary sets. Two examples of complementary muscle sets are the biceps/triceps set, and the hamstrings/quadriceps set. In a complementary set, one muscle is in full contraction, while its complement is in full extension.

Strengthening these complementary muscle sets evenly will keep your body musculature in balance and help avoid injury. Approach your exercise program with an attitude of allowing and having fun! As you do your relaxing and stretching, stretch and extend your muscles to their full range of motion (or as far as you are able). Each time you stretch and relax, you will find you are a bit more flexible and a bit more able. Pay attention to your balance, keeping your body and consciousness centered as you do your exercise, noticing how centered you are, how even and aligned your body is as it exercises. Pay attention to the refinements. For example, do you use one arm more powerfully or stronger in relationship to the other arm when doing a push-up? When walking or riding a bicycle (or stationary bike), does one leg do more work than the other? If so, you may want to consider strengthening the weaker one a bit more! Paying attention to your forward and backward movements, your side-to-side movements, and your twisting movements, you will begin to observe areas where movement, balance, and strength can be improved.

There is an idea that exercise has to be tough and painful, which is just not true. If you go as far as you can go each time you do an exercise, you will find that gradually at the perfect pace you will increase your ability in every area. The secret is just keep going, week after week, month after month, year after year. A year from now (mark your calendar), as you have continued doing this program, you will be an entirely new person; where it might have been difficult to walk two miles, you can now walk six or more with ease! Where it was hard to do even one or two push-ups, you can now do fifty, eighty, or more! Where you may have gotten winded just walking a mile or two, or just doing a bit of exercise, you now do it all with relative ease!

I of course am hoping you take your life on as a VIP—very important project! I hope you are doing directed breathing and are a master of relaxed breathing (chapter 1), becoming perfectly balanced every time you do this important life-giving exercise. I hope you are drinking distilled water, at least one glass every morning, and that you have found a good source of pure drinking water, and have a water filtration/purification system or portable home water distiller and are using it. I hope you have installed a portable air-washing unit in your home or the room of the house in which you spend the most time, and that you have found a pure-air area to live in and are living there! If you are not, I hope you are using my suggestions for spray bottle misting, and ionizers. If you have done all suggested things, great; you are probably experiencing the benefit on a daily basis. If not, on to what is next, and I invite you to consider where you have not started yet and start now! See bibliography for more information.

CHAPTER 6

Simplify, Adjust Your Use and Consumption

Start perhaps by realizing that most people consume far more than they need! Let's start with food. It is not unreasonable to state that the majority of people in the United States (and some other parts of the world) eat four to ten times more than they need or than their body requires. Those of you who eat just what you need, great. To those who do not have enough to eat, I sincerely apologize. Perhaps if I consume less, there may be more for you.

For years, I have fasted one day each week, drinking only water, not eating anything for twenty-four hours. Here is what I can share about that experience. Once your body gets trained, anywhere from three days to three months (it varies per individual), and your body becomes accustomed to the routine, instead of being hungry or worrying about food, your body just goes, "Oh, we're not eating today, no problem." Now if you normally eat 1,500 to 2,500 calories per day, and you don't eat one day per week, fifty-two weeks per year, that is an unconsumed volume of 78,000 to 130,000 calories per year! That is a lot. Boy howdy is that a lot! A funny thing happens when you fast one day a week. After your body becomes accustomed to it (three months or twelve to thirteen weeks), the day after you fast, you are not as hungry. You begin to think about and be naturally drawn to eating healthier and less food! Now some people cannot just start fasting one day a week and have it be healthy or even possible for them. You first have to honestly look at what you are eating and make an honest determination if you are consuming more than you need. Then consider reducing your daily calorie consumption by 30 to 40 percent. This will result in a weight reduction of approximately one pound per month, and if you keep at it, you can adjust your body weight by this alone. Once your weight is in a fairly healthy range, you can take on other disciplines if you desire. A good hint is if you are overweight for your height and age, you are probably consuming more than you need.

It is desirable to adjust our overall use and consumption in as many ways as we possibly can. One area for reduction can be in the amount of fuel or gasoline we use to accomplish our daily tasks. Consider eliminating your car in favor of walking and public transportation. "Did you say eliminate my car! Are you crazy! Ah!" Yes, repeat after me, "Yes, it is okay for me to eliminate my car! Yes, it is okay for me to eliminate my car! Yes, it is okay for me to eliminate my car!" In some areas, it works quite well, such as in New York, Paris, San Francisco, or any city or town where they have had the insight to install a good transit system. If you live in the right place, under the right conditions, you may be able to do this most anywhere! Consider the following: Live close to where you work (within walking distance). Live close to services and sources, organic growers and farms, and stores that carry the materials, food, and products that you may need on a day-to-day basis. Living without a vehicle can result in the following savings: You will save the cost of fuel. If you would normally drive 10,000 to 20,000 miles per year at a fuel economy of twenty-five miles per gallon of gas, that adds up to a savings of 400 to 800 gallons of gas per year or at $3.50 per gallon; that's between $1,400 and $2,800 per year savings on gas alone. Of course fuel prices fluctuate. The lowest savings is the equivalent of a weekend vacation at a reasonable place of your choice each year. The larger savings amount is enough to pay for a one-week vacation every year! Or feed 1,400 to 2,800 people one meal for a day. Or feed fourteen to twenty-eight people one meal a day for over three months! Also, you are not paying insurance, so you are saving $1,200 to $3,000 a year. And of course you are not paying maintenance, so you can save $160 per year on oil changes you don't need and $600 per year on tires you don't need, which is another $760 per year. There are also miscellaneous parts or repairs—let's say $25 per month minimum for a total of $300 per year, which added to the above is $1,060 per year. If you total the above and add in the ongoing cost of a car payment, which many people have, of $130 dollars to $300 dollars per month, that's $1,560 to $3,600 per year, and a total of $5,220 to $10,460 per year is the probable cost of owning a vehicle. Or, we could take a one-month vacation each year. Or, we could use that money to feed fourteen to twenty-eight starving people one meal a day for a year! So by not owning a car for one year, we do not have the cost of it, and we also reduce air pollution. We significantly increase our free capital and our ability to contribute to expanded opportunities for ourselves and others!

Another area we can consider adjusting our consumption is in the clothing area. Most of us own far more clothes than we need or than we can even reasonably manage. I can hear it now! "What! Give up some of my clothes? Argh! Are you crazy? I need a new ..." Here again, for those of you who need clothes or don't have more clothes than you need, I apologize to you, and if I use less, perhaps you will have more. For those of you that are clotheshorses and just really need those ten to fifty suits, and fifty to a hundred shirts, and a hundred pair of shoes, and sixty sets of underwear, and a hundred pairs of socks, I also apologize to you. Please carry on and enjoy. I still love you! If you are an average male, you probably don't need more than four suits with four to eight dress shirts, four pairs of casual dress slacks with four to eight casual shirts, and four pairs of outdoor work or recreation pants with six to eight work or recreation shirts. In addition, fourteen pairs of underwear and fourteen pairs of socks divided into dress, casual dress, and work or recreation should do it for your wardrobe. Add four to six ties for more formal wear, and four belts, a light jacket, and a heavy jacket, and that should do it. You will also need six pairs of shoes, two for dress, two for casual dress, and two for recreation or working. For women, a similar breakdown can work for clothes as well. Here again, I can hear the well-dressed women of the world going, "Are you crazy!" Well, perhaps. At least give some consideration to the positive intent of these ramblings—please, pretty please? While men and women can do with considerably less, consider two sets of dress clothes, the number of work clothes of course depends on the type of job/career you have, and two sets of casual dress outdoor play/work clothes, with underwear and accessories. Most people will want the flexibility of the items in the volume noted above. If you have more than the above noted items, you may be working with more than you need and more than may be logistically practical. Consider eliminating everything else by giving away to friends or donating your excess items. If you own two sets of dress clothes and two sets of work/recreation type clothes, you can clean one suit or one set of work/recreation type clothes while you are wearing the other set. If they are the correct material, you can hand wash the clothes and air and sun-dry them, ironing if needed. If you have the four sets of dress, casual, and work/recreation clothes, you can either hand wash each set as it becomes dirty, or you can machine wash when you have a group of four to six sets of clothes that need cleaning, ironing if needed. If it is necessary to send clothes to a dry cleaner, use one that uses nontoxic cleaning material.

If we have adjusted our consumption over the last pages, we are spending considerably less money and finding ourselves with considerably more flexibility and organization, physically and mentally, with a variety of options and choices before us. The next area to consider adjusting our consumption is in the variable personal choices we make on a day-to-day basis. Do we really need those three or four extra gourmet coffees per week at a cost of fifteen to twenty dollars a week? (Here, in the interest of full disclosure, I want to tell you I love a good cup of coffee, and I am not suggesting you eliminate coffee, just those three or four extra gourmet coffees per week). Or that ice cream or pastry, which is not good for us anyway, at a cost of five dollars to fifteen or more per week? Can we instead of going out to eat and spending twenty dollars or more for dinner, stay home and save twenty dollars per week? So let's say we can save about forty to fifty-five dollars per person per week (coffee, pastry, eating out). For a family of three, that would be $120 to $165 per week, a fairly significant amount. If you figure the savings in a year (for that family of three), it is $6,240 to $8,580 per year. That would be a significant level of savings! Smart choices in many other areas yield considerable savings on housing, energy consumption, water, electric and gas bills, paper, printing, office supplies, and personal purchases. Considering the intent and adoption of practices related to our previous conversations, it should be fairly simple to identify and figure out how to reduce consumption in these areas as well.

CHAPTER 7

Environmental Living

Make life-supportive choices. Consider everything we buy, wear, use, live in, eat, or play with, in the context of environmental living. Environmental living is actually living in a way that maximizes the health and well-being of every living thing on the planet and supports life in general, including ours! Everything from the soaps we buy to the products we buy and the types of packages the stuff we buy comes in. Also, the types of materials and products we use have an effect on our environment.

Walking is healthier and more life supporting than driving. Here I make a statement relating to our lifestyle and the effect it has on our environment. We live in a remarkably interconnected environment.

Everything we do has an impact on something else. I encourage you to begin by not using anything such as pesticide, herbicide, or germicide. No matter what anyone says, these products are very harmful to humans and other living things. They wind up in our air, our water, and our body tissues and in no way support our health.

Nature has developed in such a way that it is always working at balancing itself, and if we do not artificially intercede, nature does the most efficient and effective job possible in this regard. Our interconnected world is an amazingly design-efficient system if we let it occur naturally! For this part, each of us has to think about what our commitment to the environment is and what we are willing to do to protect it, to have a healthier, happier world. Here are some thoughts and suggestions to consider. Support and foster the growth of life-supportive businesses such as local organic growers and businesses that support life-affirming systems. Use natural products in your home and buy them from responsible sources. Use biodegradable and healthy life-supporting cleaning products. Buy in bulk wherever possible (health-food stores, some health-oriented supermarkets, etc.). Use your own containers or buy things that are in biodegradable and people-safe containers. Paper and glass are generally people supportive, and plastic is not. Filling your own clean glass container or paper bag from a bulk food bin is much better than buying food in a separate container that then becomes waste. If the container you buy is plastic, it then becomes a problem causing waste because most plastic is not biodegradable and can be toxic to process as well.

It is safe to say that each of our daily choices is either supporting our life or harming us and others, and it is up to us to take closer looks at these daily choices and make those choices that protect and sustain life. Make your dollars work protecting you, all of us, and the environment by investing in responsible, socially and environmentally sensible business. Our daily choices can and will protect and sustain all our lives, if we choose wisely.

Another area of wise environmental choice is clothing and various fabric-related purchases. Here consider using sustainable, life-supporting, naturally grown and processed fabrics such as, cotton, silk, wool, linen, bamboo, and paper, which are generally life supporting and healthier to use and wear. In general, look in every area of your life and make product selections based on life affirming choices. Think in terms of, which choices are the very best environmental choices here? If you truly don't know, do a little research, use the Internet, and ask people engaged in environmentally responsible activities, such as organic gardeners or farmers, or heirloom seed growers, or naturopathic doctors, or natural scientists, nutritionists, or herbalists. Then make those wise, informed choices. In a world where everything is related, all of our choices have an effect; we affect everyone else whether we see it or not. See the bibliography for more information.

CHAPTER 8

Body Cleansing, the Schley Skin Brushing System, and Fasting

Complete body cleansing occurs faster, more fully, and healthier with pure air, pure water, pure organically grown, non-GMO, non-irradiated, nontoxic, locally grown food and good exercise. When we begin to cleanse our body inside and outside, in our own interest we need to keep the messages of the previous chapters in mind! Let us start with the outside of our body. There are different people with different skin types and different needs. There are people with sensitive skin, moderately sensitive skin, and skin that is not sensitive. There are people with oily skin, moderately oily skin, and people with dry skin. Some people have allergic reactions to different substances, and most of you probably are aware of the type of skin you have and its sensitivity level. There are general rules that everyone can use and that generally work well for everyone.

Rule #1

Live the first four chapters of this book to the best of your ability.

Rule #2

Stay away from the "antis" and the "cides," including bactericide. If it's "antis" or "cides," stay away from it to live healthy and well. Antis include antibacterial soaps, antiperspirant, and antibiotics, to name a few. You know some of the "cides" are automatically not good for you, like suicide, homicide, pesticide, and herbicide. Just stay away from all of them to be safe. With the cides, you are killing something, and the antis are automatically against something. Ultimately, if we are killing something or against something, it always comes back to us sooner or later!

Rule #3

Use only natural, toxic-free, chemical-free, pure air, water, food, and healthy healing products on and in your body and at home to keep it naturally clean. Avoid antiperspirant. Most antiperspirants block the natural elimination of the skin, the free function of which is essential for optimal health. Sweat or perspiration does not have a bad odor in the healthy body. It is a natural process, and if you lead a really healthy life, your sweat or perspiration does not have a bad odor, though it can make you damp or wet. The message is stay away from anti products as much as you possibly can, or use as little as possible. Use products that are as natural as possible so as not to interfere with the natural elimination processes of the body.

The goal of true cleansing is to encourage the flow of toxic materials out of the body, not to stop the flow, as in antiperspirant. I repeat that the goal is to encourage the natural cleansing flow of toxic materials out of the body, not to suppress them.

Consider making your own cleansers and soaps out of organic, natural, healthy, healing materials. These cleansers, lotions, soaps, or oils can be tailored specifically to you and can really give you a wonderful and magical all-natural, healthy, healing cleaning experience. Your own mini spa at home daily! You can of course have these made for you if you look around, and you can also find excellent already-made products that are natural and good for you as well. We should say here that if you have suppressed skin elimination in some way, there may be a period of time where your skin eliminates more than usual, which is the body's way of catching up on its elimination duties. Once it has done this and balanced out, optimal skin health can result.

Schley Skin Brushing System

The next topic for body cleansing is the Schley Skin Brushing System. For this, you can use a vegetable bristle brush with a long detachable handle so you can reach those harder-to-reach places on the body like your back. You can also use a vegetable sponge like loofa; however, I prefer the vegetable bristle brush. The Schley Skin Brushing System should be used with common sense; do not use on wounds, sensitive or injured skin, or on skin conditions where fungal or other kinds of conditions could be transferred to other parts of the body. Check with your physician or health care professional before using this system if you have any questions regarding your skin condition. See the illustrations on the following two pages (front of the body and back of the body) that illustrate the flow of the brushing. Read the directions that follow the illustrations and then use the Schley Skin Brushing System.

1. **Schley Skin Brushing System** **4.**

SKIN	**BRUSH FROM**
BRUSH	**TOES TO**
FRONT	**HEELS ON**
BODY	**BOTTOM**
FROM	**OF FEET,**
CHEST	**UP**
DOWN	**INSIDE**
INSIDE	**FRONT**
ARMS TO	**OF LEGS,**
HANDS AND	**TORSO, AND**
OUT FINGERS	**CHEST**

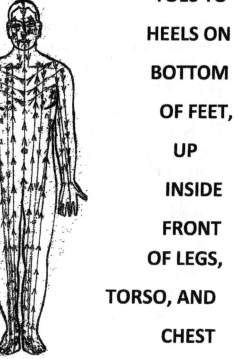

Schley Skin Brushing System

Front Body

3. **Schley Skin Brushing System** **2.**

FROM TOP		**BRUSH**
OF HEAD	Schley Skin Brushing System	**FINGERS**
DOWN NECK,		**UP BACK**
SHOULDERS		**OF HANDS**
TORSO AND		**ARMS**
LOWER BACK		**OVER**
BUTTOCKS		**SHOULDERS**
THIGHS, LEGS		**AND NECK**
OUTSIDE CALVES		**FACE**
OVER TOP OF		**AND**
FEET AND		**TOP**
OUT TOES		**OF HEAD**

Back Body

Brush your whole body in the number sequence 1, 2, 3, 4, shown on the two facing pages. You will notice that number 1 is on the Front Body illustration, and number 2 is on the Back Body illustration. Number 3 is also on the Back Body illustration, and number 4 is on the Front Body illustration. The brushing flow is front, back, back, front, and you repeat the sequence a total of three full times. Front, back, back, front, front, back, back, front, front, back, back, front. The pattern is consistent with the flow of energy in the meridians of your body, which flow in an alternating yin, yang, yang, yin sequence. The sequence repeated three times—yin, yang, yang, yin, yin, yang, yang, yin, yin, yang, yang, yin—holds a secret related to the flow of energy in the universe and our holographic body. This flow helps balance and strengthen the body energy field, stimulates body circulation and lymphatic flow, and promotes body and skin cleansing at deeper levels. Take your long-handled vegetable bristle body brush and begin dry skin brushing in the following pattern, starting with number 1. Imagine your nude body, your head facing forward, your right hand in a comfortable position palm forward, your left hand in a comfortable position palm forward, your right foot pointing comfortably to the right, and your left foot pointing comfortably to the left; we will refer to this as the front body and inside of your body. On the front side, you have the front of your head, your chest and torso, the inside, sides, and front of your arms, and the inside, sides, and front of your legs.

The back body is the back of your head, the back of your chest and torso, and the back, outside, and sides of your arms, and the back, outside, and sides of your legs, essentially accounting for the rest of the body. Start with the Front Body illustration. Start dry skin brushing with number 1, and with the brush in your right hand, start at the center chest. Brush from the center chest, down the inside and sides of the left arm, palm and hand, and out the fingers. Then put the brush in your left hand and brush your skin from the center chest, down the inside and sides of the right arm, palm and hand, and out the ends of the fingers. This was step 1 (front body).

Keeping the brush in your left hand, do step number 2 (back body). Brush up the outside of fingers and back of right hand, outside arm, over the top and outside of your shoulder, up your neck, the side and right half of your face to the top of your head. Then put the brush in your right hand, brush up the outside back of your fingers and the back of your left hand and arm, over the top and the outside of your left shoulder, up your neck, the side and left half of your face to the top of your head. This was step number 2 (back body). Now step number 3 (back body). You may need to add the brush handle to allow you to reach down your back. Brush from the top and sides of your head down the back and outside of your head, neck, and shoulders. Continue down the back of your torso, down the back and sides of your buttocks, legs, and out the top outside of your feet and toes, making sure you cover both left and right sides thoroughly. This was step number 3 (back body). Next is step number 4 (front body). With the brush in your right hand, starting at the toes of your left foot, brush the bottom of the foot to the heel, and bottom inside of the foot, and up the inside sides and front of the left leg, up the front inside and sides of your hips, abdomen, and torso, up to the chest. Then put the brush in your left hand and, starting at the toes of the right foot, brush the bottom of the foot to the heel, and bottom inside and sides of the foot, and up the inside sides and front of the right leg, up the front inside and sides of your hips, abdomen, and torso, up to your chest. This was step 4 (front body).

This completes one 1, 2, 3, 4, cycle. Repeat all the brushing sequences two more times. After doing the three times, imagine a center body line starting between your legs and going up the front of the body to just below the lower lip line, going inside through your tongue pressed to the roof of your mouth, then going outside to the center of your upper lip just below your nose, up the center of your face, over the top of the head, and down the center of the neck, back, and torso to the starting point at the center of the body between the legs. Imagine this connecting the body energy. Then reverse the flow going up the back to the top of the head, down the face center line to the upper lip just below the nose, inside to the roof of the mouth, connecting to the tongue (which is pressed to the roof of the mouth), down the tongue and out to just below the lower lip line, down the center of the chin, neck, torso, to the starting point at the center of the body between the legs. Repeat three times, finishing with going up the center line to the mouth with the tongue pressed to the roof of your mouth.

Congratulations! You have completed one full Schley Skin Brushing System cycle and centering. It sounds complicated, but once you have done it, the entire dry skin brushing and centering can be done in less than ten minutes. The net effect of skin brushing is healthier skin, improved circulation of blood and lymph, and a stimulated and balanced energy field. I suggest that dry skin brushing not be used more frequently than every four days, and if your skin gets tender, you may have to allow an additional two or three days for the skin to balance out. This will allow the benefits of the session to fully integrate with the body systems. I personally feel amazingly alert, energized, and balanced after doing skin brushing. I suggest taking a short shower rinse off after skin brushing with cool and then cold water (or as cool as you can for a few minutes). Do not dry your body; just put on a clean (preferably natural fiber) robe and let your body heat flush the skin surface and dry your body.

Once you have done this, you will understand its value. Treat your body and your skin as a precious resource that deserves to be naturally pampered with natural, healthy, healing, nourishing cleaners, oils, and lotions. You deserve it.

Fasting

For the internal body cleansing process, we need to start by choosing what we are going to consume more carefully. As discussed in chapters 3 and 4, whichever eating style you have chosen, be sure your food is organically grown, toxin-free, healthy, natural, and preferably locally grown. If you eat beef, it should be organically grown, free range, and certified with no antibiotics or hormones. Chickens should be free range, naturally organically grown and fed. Fish should be wild caught, not introduced species, and not farmed species grown with antibiotics and chemicals, and colorings. Grains and beans may be added as needed.

Let's proceed with internal cleansing. As with any of the processes suggested in this book, if you have any question or concerns, please consult your physician or natural health care professional to determine if you are able to proceed.

If you are serious about obtaining optimal health, you might consider fasting one day per week, and doing a three-and-a-half-day fasting and cleansing process twice a year. This is best done on or near the equinoxes and solstices. You might include such a program in your life now. I suggest you make a one-year commitment to consume only natural healthy food and pure water, and to breathe as healthy air as possible. I suggest that you also commit to a regular exercise program for this year, generally using this book's exercise information and healthy living chapters as a guide. I also suggest you consider doing two liver flushes during the course of this year, preferably one at the spring equinox and one at the summer solstice. I also suggest you consider doing two enemas or colonics. A good time is on or near the spring equinox and on or near the summer solstice.

This will help ease toxic material out of the body. As with any of the suggestions in this book, if you have any question or concerns, please consult a natural health care professional or your physician to determine if you are able to proceed. Unless you have fasted quite a bit in your life, I do not recommend beginning with more than a three-and-a-half-day fasting process. When you have done the one healthy year recommended, including the two liver flushes and two enemas or colonics, and you are not taking over-the-counter or prescription medications, you may consider adopting an additional once or twice a year natural fasting process. This process consists of beginning a fast and continuing it until your hunger returns. When fasting, it is essential to have a pure water source. Use distilled water for half of your total water consumption, best consumed starting in the morning, with your first thing consumed being eight to twelve ounces of water. Pure, spring, new, or artesian water may be used for the other half of your fasting water. If you do not have access to pure, spring, new, or artesian water, use whatever pure or filtered water you are confident in for the other half of your daily water consumption.

Fasting like everything else is cyclic. If you wish to see a graphic representation of your body and its cleansing process, you can assemble eight to fourteen glass jars with lids and put them somewhere convenient to your bathroom, and during your fasting process, I suggest you save your urine each day in these jars, numbering or dating the jars one to fourteen. At the end of your fasting, you will have a tool that will allow you to visually observe the elimination process your body goes through during fasting. You will find that the urine starts out whatever color it is, and as the fast goes on, the urine gets progressively denser. Save all urine samples. Put the jars you saved in one place for a few days to a week, and look at them on the third day and the eighth day after your fast. What you will see is a memorable graphic indicator of the progress of your fast.

It is entirely possible that for every day we fast, we get an additional day of life! The longest I have fasted is fourteen days. I have known people who have fasted longer. I do not believe that fasting longer is better. I believe that moderation in all things is desirable, and therefore I believe that three and a half days, seven days, or fourteen days are generally ideal approximate fasting durations. Shorter fasts may be used, unless you have a specific physical, spiritual, emotional, or medical intention. If that is your intention, I suggest you find a responsible professional to assist you in these areas, unless you have a great deal of experience and are confident of your own knowledge and ability.

My own experiences and my experiences of listening to and observing friends who have fasted for various purposes leads me to express that I know fasting can be used to heal the body, mind, and spirit, and I encourage you to do some experiencing on your own so that you have the experience!

Any one of these topics can be a book of its own, but if you take the information on body cleansing to heart and follow the suggested directions, you will experience success. A short note here in relation to over-the-counter or prescription medication. I support natural healing processes and the use of natural methods of healing, which does not include anything that is not organic, natural, or energetically balancing. Using naturally derived supplements, herbs, oils, cleansers, and natural healing systems such as massage therapy, chiropractors, naturopaths, herbalists, applied kinesiology, and other natural health systems, in my opinion, is the only way to go! Many people in the healing arts have adopted natural health practices because they have found that supporting the body's natural healing processes just works better. If you or someone you know has a serious accident or other life-threatening mechanical body damage, please go straight to a hospital and let the medical profession put you back together, as our technology is really very good at that. As in previous chapters of this book, I refer you to the bibliography at the end of this book to assist you in your ongoing adventure!

CHAPTER 9

Health, Color, and Healing

What is health and healing? The words are derived from hale or whole. The general condition of health is described as of body and mind, with reference to soundness and vigor. Healing is described as the act or process of being whole, usually experienced as freedom from pain, illness, anxiety, and so on. This freedom is experienced as the ease of functioning of body, mind, and spirit. Health is wholeness, and healing is the act or process of being whole.

We all come from the light. We are light physically expressed. We all return to the light, and our soul is expressed as light. Our being and our physical body consist of a series of harmonic and complementary rainbow bridges. If you are a fan of health, color, and healing and would like access to the holographic body and the universal holographic database and you have studied some of these subjects and their relation to life and health, then this chapter is for you. If you don't care for these subjects, you could skip this chapter, but by reading it, you just might discover something.

We are all light. This comes from my study of color, health, healing, muscle testing, energy, meditation, and the holographic body. As you read in the beginning of this book, we all began as a soul merging with the physical, as sperm/ovum, united with a flash of blue light, holoprinting, the holographic matrix of the universe and genetic structure, beginning the nine-month holoprinting process in the holoprinter (mom). We then emerge into our apparently three-dimensional world. Now, I have not personally seen this flash of blue light that prints the holoprint pattern of the holographic matrix of the universe. For this information, I thank the late Dr. Marcel Vogel (holder of a great number of patents, the father of liquid crystalline displays and a crystal expert) for his description during a workshop I attended years ago. I do remember asking him, "You actually physically saw this flash of blue light as the sperm/ovum united?" To which he replied, "Yes." From my own study, I am sure that our universe and we are kept in place by a holographic matrix of light harmonic frequencies that are simply intricate and intricately simple.

Colors are our experience of different energy frequencies. We have an accepted language of color in which much of our color reality is expressed—"red as a beet," "green with envy" or jealousy, "feeling gray," "feeling blue," a "golden touch," "yellow-bellied coward," "purple with rage," "indigo mood," "feeling in the pink," and many more. Color awareness can help us understand our experiences, create them, and enhance our lives. By shifting our color relationships in life, we can shift our reality and our experiences. By being aware of our color reality, we can access valuable information for every part of our life.

Have you ever wondered why the vast majority of fast-food businesses have combinations of advertising colors that all, predominately, together, or individually, feature the color orange? Would it interest you to know that the color orange is directly related to our body energy system? Food as a carrier of this energy, our digestive system as a processor of this energy, our sense of smell as a sensor, our basic energy (known as Life Force, Prana, Chi, Ki), our breathing, and whether or not we are comfortable socially—they all are directly related to the color orange. A brief insight into this relationship is that the color orange stimulates the stomach meridian. The stomach processes the food we consume that ultimately becomes the fuel our body uses, and anyone who has built a campfire recognizes orange as a dominant color of burning fuel. This fuel along with our breathing supports our basic energy (known as Life Force, Prana, Chi, and Ki). Orange, highly visible, and getting attention, is an extroverts color. When a major bank "changed its colors," shifting its branding logo from then traditional "banker's blue" to a dominant almost fast-food red-orange logo, I remember predicting the shift and ultimate demise of that banking system as we knew it. When the bank initially saw a rise in success and profit, I thought the bank's approach to our gut-level, visceral, basic energy (red-orange, fast-food) system must have succeeded. Today we can all realize that the bank traded the safer, traditional, more conservative, constant and predictable system for the vagaries of gut-level, visceral, highly mutable, instant gratification. Think many trillions of dollars, an ultimately dangerous financial system. Much like trading a locally, organically grown GMO-free, healthy food system for a continuous factory-farmed, mass-produced, and manufactured fast-food system. We get "full" initial satisfaction at what may wind up being a very expensive long-term cost! Getting back to color, the examples used clearly show the color relationships to our daily lives, and more importantly, they are concrete indicators of the premise of this chapter, which is that we are all light. An in-depth understanding of color in our world will provide us with a key to understanding our holographic body, where the smallest part of the body is actually an energetic blueprint of the entire body. "In as much as ye have done it to the least of these my children, ye have done it unto me." This biblical quote could be used when comparing and referencing the holographic body. Holy body for short! What is color living? Color living is allowing ourselves to play with and experience the greatest variety of colors in the greatest variety of circumstances possible. In the earlier food chapter, "eating a rainbow" was suggested, meaning consuming the greatest variety of healthy foods possible. Using color as an indicator provides a great variety of nutritional and health benefits. The idea is that color is a major indicator informing our life! Do you love fashion? Have you consulted a fashion color consultant? Have you checked out what fashion colors work the best for you? Do you love art? Are you an artist? Would you like to be an artist and use color as a means of self-expression? Do you love color? Are your clothes, your home, and your life an expression of your love of color? Would you like to learn a failsafe system to find out what colors are great for you personally or for anyone you know? Would you like to learn how to best use color everywhere in your life? If so, read on! Color is a major indicator informing our life, and learning a system to find out what colors are good for us personally, or anyone, and how best to use color everywhere or anywhere in life is a valuable tool. We begin by realizing that our body is a part of a universal holographic system, within which all information is contained, and that access to this information is always available, much like accessing your cloud-stored information, your files on a computer, or looking up files in a file cabinet, only the database is universal and holographic. Our bodies function as a universal holographic interactive database where all information can be accessed. Those of you familiar with muscle testing or applied kinesiology have already been using this body information system to determine muscle strength and weakness, and with your knowledge of the body systems and muscle, meridian, acupressure, massage, and organ-related systems, you are able to help someone balance their own body based on the indicator muscle's strength or weakness. One important value of muscle testing in my opinion is its application with people where they can personally and directly experience the validation of what is "true" and will contribute to their wholeness, health, and well-being, indicated by a strong test. Another value is directly experiencing what is "not true," indicated by a not strong muscle test, what will not contribute to their wholeness, health, and well-being at this time.

Here is the muscle testing process. Two people, one who is doing the muscle testing (the tester) and one who is being tested, stand in relation to each other in a way that is convenient for the tester to muscle test the person being tested. The tester selects the muscle to be tested and asks permission of the person being tested if it is okay with them to do the muscle testing. If it is okay, the selected muscle is "tested in the clear" to determine that the muscle being tested is strong. The muscle testing process is not a contest of strength; it is a process where the tester, using the minimum amount of pressure possible, determines if a muscle is "strong." This is determined when the muscle being tested "holds" against the pressure being used by the tester. A typical muscle test is done by the person being tested extending their arm in front of or to the side of their body. My preference is the arm forward and rotated so the thumb is in a downward position. The tester placing two fingers on the arm behind the wrist and gently but firmly pushes downward, while the job of the person being tested is to maintain the muscle position. One of two things will happen; either the muscle locks and does not go downward with the pressure (a strong test, "true" test) or the muscle does not lock, and the arm moves downward, apparently not able to "hold" (a not strong, "not true" test). If the muscle is strong "true" test, then you have a muscle you can use for muscle testing. If the muscle is not strong, a "not true "test, and we are testing in the clear, this is an indication of an energy block, indicated by muscle weakness. We must then either help the person being tested strengthen the muscle or choose a different muscle that tests strong. People with applied kinesiology or muscle testing training can usually help a person balance the body, which then results in strong muscle testing.

If you do not have this training, then please find a different muscle that tests strong in the clear. There is no "kind of a strong test." The muscle is strong and locks—or it is not strong and does not lock. A bouncy muscle is also a "not strong" test. This muscle testing procedure is best accomplished in a quiet, neutral environment, with no music or other distractions. If the person being tested stands against a table or next to a chair, they could close their eyes to eliminate any visual distractions, although this is not generally necessary. This muscle testing process can also be done if the person is seated or lying on a massage, chiropractic, or examining table, in which case the pressure of the test on an outstretched arm would be directed toward the feet. It is also possible to use any strong muscle for testing, in which case the test is holding the muscle at the middle of its range of motion and testing that the muscle locks or does not lock when pressure is applied in the direction of the range of motion.

When I say you can ask any question in muscle testing that is exactly what I mean. I consider it advisable to get the permission of the person being tested for the general subject area of the testing, as a professional courtesy, and both people should be authentically engaged in the inquiry. The only muscle testing requirement is that the questions must be in the form of a statement able to be answered by a yes or true (strong test), or a no or not true (not strong test). This muscle testing procedure gives you and the person being tested direct access to the holographic body and the universal holographic database, which contains all information. With practice, like anything else, one will improve and become more proficient at asking questions and receiving answers.

The physical body has developed over centuries, millennia, and in fact has developed sensory systems that cause us to move toward that which is good for us, (yes) a strong muscle test, and away from that which is not good for us, (no) a not strong muscle test. It is this usually subconscious system that gives us access through the holographic body to the universal holographic database. It is helpful if both the person doing the muscle testing and the person being tested are willing to do the tests, are neutral, and are generally supportive of the inquiry. The only limit to muscle testing that I am aware of is that muscle testing cannot be used to predict the future. It can, however, give us current-time information related to the future and assist us in creating the future, if that is an area of interest. As noted earlier, if you find a muscle that tests "not strong" in the clear, it is an indication of an energy block in the physical body. There are ways to help people strengthen these muscles and balance their bodies, using the information contained in this book, and one can even ask the body the best way to balance a muscle and the body energy if you like, using a strong body muscle for the tests. There are a number of different ways to conduct muscle tests. One way is to verbally make a statement, such as, "Vitamin C is good for (state the name of the person being tested)." Then muscle test with a strong test being a yes, and a not strong test being a no. Another way is to hold the item being tested in contact with the body of the person being tested; a strong test indicating what is being tested is good for the person, and a not strong test indicating what is not good for the person. It is important to determine the amount of anything someone intends to take internally, and the period of time to take that amount (for example, one teaspoon three times per day, for four days). A convenient place to hold the item being tested is at the solar plexus level either in the front or back of the body. The interesting thing about this test is that the body will test accurately and respond to the item being tested whether or not the individual or the tester knows what the items are (blind test). The reason for this is, as noted early on, we are all light or harmonic frequencies of light, and we are all swimming so to speak in the same light energy soup, and when we bring something close to us or in contact with us, it influences our soup, so to speak, and we get a holographic field test in the moment. In my opinion, there is no more comprehensive test than this. Everything in the universe has a frequency rate, and our sensory systems can sense that rate and whether or not the item being tested strengthens us and is good for us (true/yes) or does not strengthen us and is not good for us (not true / no). When a number of muscle tests have been done, depending on the individual, the muscle being tested may tend to fatigue, at which time one must discontinue the tests or select an alternative strong muscle for testing while the fatigued muscle rests and rebalances. Earlier in this chapter, I promised you access to color information, and here it is. Using the muscle testing procedure, any color in any form can be tested in proximity to or against your body, or on the wall, or in your environment to determine if the color item is good for you at that location. I have found that it can be beneficial if a person who is being tested for colors they are going to wear does not know what color is being tested, as more tests can be done rapidly before the person being tested reaches a fatigued state. Use color swatches held at the back at the solar plexus level and then test yes/no, rapidly going through as many colors as desired at a sitting. It is good to consider that color can be an individual thing, and in areas where several people are going to be living, all the color preferences should be considered, coming up with colors for a shared environment that are harmonic, or complementary, with the greatest number of people.

In addition to muscle testing another, valuable tool is scanning. The following are definitions of scanning.

1. To examine the particulars or to scrutinize
2. To glance at or over, to read hastily, as in to scan a page
3. To observe repeatedly or sweepingly, a minute or large expanse
4. As in medical biology, to examine a body, organ, tissue, or other biologically active material with a scanner

The definition of a scanner is a person or machine that scans. When we shop, most stores have mechanical scanners that read and enter the price of your items in the shop's computer. When we scan, we become the scanner. Anyone can learn how to scan. I have taught scanning to kids and adults. Scanning is like everything else in the world, available to us as we learn, practice, and use ourselves as scanners. There are as many different methods to scan and be scanners as we can imagine. Here is one system I use when shopping for or choosing food, supplements, or anything that I will use for myself or my family. The first step is to define what you are looking for or want. As an example, food or supplements of optimal value for my health (items of optimal value may change, so be sure to recheck periodically).

Next, go to where there is a concentration of what you seek. In the case of food or supplements, that may be a healthy-food Store, co-op, organic farm, or farmers' market. Now, state your intention and how your intention will occur. For example, "I will use my hand to scan the food or supplements available. My hand will automatically stop at the food or supplements that are of optimal value, right now, to my health." Then, begin scanning with your hand slowly moving across the items being scanned until your hand stops. Some people will be able to do this instantly, and for some it will take some practice to perfect this process. It is possible that a different form of experience may apply to different individuals, such as instead of your hand stopping, you feel an energy increase or boost, or some variation that applies to you, such as a smooth feeling or a knowing sense at a certain spot. Learn to trust yourself and to check on your results with experience. Ultimately you will be able to scan with 100 percent accuracy! Visual scanning by humans can exceed the ability of optical or electronic scanners. For instance, people who work on fruit processing lines of canneries proved to be way more effective at selecting the color differences of peaches, relative to degree of ripeness, than any machine. Imagine that by using our eyes and/or our hands for sensory and visual input, we can actually read the energy transmitted from any substance.

We are the scanner!

As the scanner, we can now proceed to scan the holographic body. In this process, we will use our scanning ability to scan the human body for energy blocks. When working with people, it is advisable that we explain what the process is and how it works. The beginning process is always the same. State your intention and how your intention will occur. Define what you are looking for and want. "I will use my hand to scan the body for major and minor energy blocks. My hand will stop at the edge of any energy block. Using this scanning method, I can describe the size and location of the energy blocks in the body." For this example, we will be using the previously described system of scanning using the hand. We begin scanning with our hand moving slowly across the body of the person being scanned. When we are over an area of energy blockage, our hand will stop, as if hitting an invisible wall, or as previously mentioned, we will sense an energy difference. This difference may manifest as a decrease in energy, or an increase in temperature (cold or hot), or a tactile difference of rough or hard energy. Whatever the energy manifestation for you is, that will be the indicator for the particular thing we are looking for. In this instance, we are looking for energy blocks. By energy blocks, we mean anything that is causing difficulty or interfering with the natural holographic flow of the body energy. Another way of defining what we are looking for is to look for major central blocks and minor or peripheral blocks. This will ultimately train us to sense the major and minor holographic energy blocks in the body.

Once you have determined and noted the energy blocks, you can then, with the permission of the person involved, proceed to assist the person in clearing the energy blocks. There are many ways to assist someone in releasing energy blocks. One way I find most effective is to have the person take a deep breath through their nose and imagine that breath is going to the area where your hand is at the energy block. Then have the person exhale with the intention of allowing the block to release and for balance to occur in the blocked area. After the person has done this one to three times, you can scan the area. The majority of the time, there will no longer be an energy block at that location, and you can move on to other areas indicated by scanning. At some point, the energy blocks will have been released in the whole body, and the body will experience a holy moment or balance of the holographic body. This is one of the methods I use in assisting someone to balance and heal their body.

For further research, I refer you to the bibliography at the end of this book.

CHAPTER 10

Holographic Body Transcends the Imagining—Or Does It?

Every part of our body, even the smallest part, is actually an energetic blueprint of the entire body. Reflexology gives insight into the holographic nature of our body, in that the hands reflect the entire body, and the feet reflect the entire body. An example is hand and foot reflexology. The eyes reflect the entire body; an example is our unique eye print, or iris print, and the science of iridology. The ears reflect the entire body; an example is auricular reflexology, also known as auricular therapy. The tongue reflects the entire body, the teeth reflect the entire body, and a drop of blood reflects the entire body. An example of the blood reflecting the entire body is the process known as sensitive crystallization! Every part of the body reflects the entire body when one knows how to read it. I refer you to the bibliography at the end of this book for more information. The examples mentioned provide you with enough evidence of this relationship that you can relate to it as fact. (I have experienced the holographic body, but that is a story for another time.) Our body is uniquely ours and simultaneously comprehensively holographic. Building on our opening conversation, in the beginning of this book, we left off at birth and the beginning of our apparently three-dimensional physical existence. Immediately at birth we begin our constantly adapting growth and development, based on our experiences in our strange new world. Everything seems different! We have transitioned in a relatively short period of time from a world of being protected, warm, with heartbeat, circulation, sound, emotions, soft energy, and a liquid oriented environment to the bright, dry, air-sucking, wind-blowing, loud, open, exposed, somewhat shocking, entirely different world existence. "Here I am, born!" Consider that we have gone from what seems like nothing, an idea, a concept, to the point of conception (swimming sperm, waiting egg, soul, a flash of light, a holoprint), to an "apparently three-dimensional physical existence." You will find this reference to "apparently three-dimensional physical existence" a number of times in this text. The intent of this phrase is to remind us that all dimensions exist simultaneously and that our current existence occurs to people as only three-dimensional. We are evolving and developing in what seems to be a complex system designed for survival and the propagation of the species. Having just popped out of our holoprinting water world environment into an entirely different reality of detached nutrition, open-air breathing, and so on, it is amazing that we can function at all. Now, logically speaking, it would seem we should have the ability to go in the reverse direction, back through the water world with its attached nutrition, back to the holographic body, to the preformed physical state, back to our universal holographic matrix existence, conscious of the entire universe! This universal holographic database is where we can experience the consciousness of our lovemaking parents and continue apparently back in time if we wish. Then by reversing direction go forward into possible futures! Why not? Of course we could. When? Now! There? Here? The adventure begins! Experience the virtual reality, cellular resonance, constantly adapting. My dear friend Brother Christopher says, "If we are in our mind, we are already late to the party." When we begin with the heart, if we can conceive it and believe it, we achieve it. As a matter of fact, if we can conceive of something, it already exists; it has an ex is tence!

We are now at a point where visual aids may be helpful.

The point is—we are the holographic body, a holographic matrix. This is an illustration which attempts to show (with a few examples) that we are the point and all the expressions of the point. Imagine that the point in the illustration is a projector lens and that the holographic matrix (us and everything) is being projected through the lens, and what we see, the earth, a human being, an embryo, and a cell, are just four of the infinite projections, (possible point expressions) in our holographic universe!

THE POINT IS-

Holographic Body

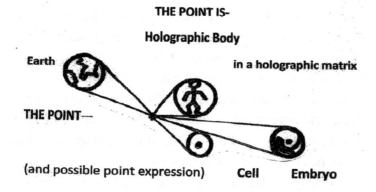

Just as a tree grows from a seed through the expansion of its holographic blueprint into our apparently three-dimensional world, so too does a human being evolve. Just as a tree grows, matures, and produces seeds, so too does every living thing produce in its likeness. Seeds seem the same and at the same time different. The moment, now, of the point of being, affects and effects being. When we know now backward and forward, we have won the present. Remember the holoprint? A flash of light and the point—existence is made. This point in the universal holographic matrix (the infinite field of our existence) is a simultaneous created response and a resonant unit or cell. "I" is created! The explanation follows. We start with a single point; we call this point a "point of focus," a "point of intent" ion into an expanded space, and we call this expanded space the infinite universe. What occurs in this infinite universe when a point of intent ion exists (apparently at the same point of conception) is that the infinite universe, designed to guarantee the survival of the matrix (us and all), responds with a duplicate image (mirror, mirror, on the wall). "I," so to speak, is created! "I am," signifying existence, is present! The following illustrations provide a visual sense of the preceding text regarding the creative principle in a dimensionally interactive reality. The point x divides and one becomes two (mirror image).

The universal holographic matrix context

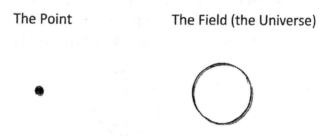

The Point   The Field (the Universe)

The point, the field (the universe)

The Point in the Field

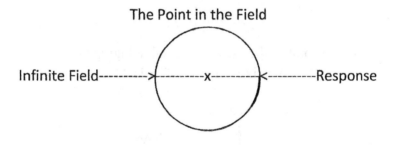

Infinite Field--------->---------x---------<---------Response

Universal holographic matrix

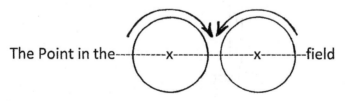

The Point in the----|------x------|------x------|--field

The point X divides and one becomes two, (mirror image).

The point in the field and universal holographic
matrix response is infinite.

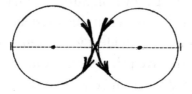

The two interact as one.

The point in the field, X marks the spot, and universal
holographic matrix response become "I" or "one."
"Where two or more gather together, there I am also."

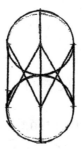

Point in the field, universal holographic
matrix is "I am," "I" x ist "I"

"I" x ist "I"

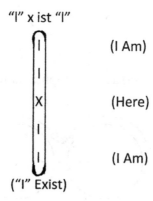

(I Am)

(Here)

(I Am)

("I" Exist)

I Am   x   Here   IST   I AM   thus   That   I Am"

I	I	(I Am)
X	X	(Here)
IST	I	(I Am)
T	T	That
H	H	I
U	U	A
S	S	M

Here I recognize that our adventure seems to be expressing itself in the form of the Greek word for fish *ixithus* or *icthyus*. I have to admit that it appears as if something is trying to express itself as holographic expression, possibly validating the story of the Christian faith relating to the fish symbol and the loaves of bread (John 6, verses 9–14).

Two fish and five loaves of bread.
We can see the fish (symbol) and the two fish
and five loaves of bread extended.

(><><) ><> <> <> <> <> <> <><

When connected, the fishes and the loaves of bread are

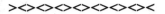

one strand of the universal holographic matrix. This strand, when stacked with other strands, can be represented as a physical graph or chart that applies to all humanity.

The next page shows a black and white universal holographic matrix illustration surrounded by some sacred symbols that are all part of the universal holographic matrix.

A color version of this universal holographic matrix
is on the front and back cover of this book.

THE "UNIVERSAL HOLOGRAPHIC MATRIX"

And Sacred Symbols

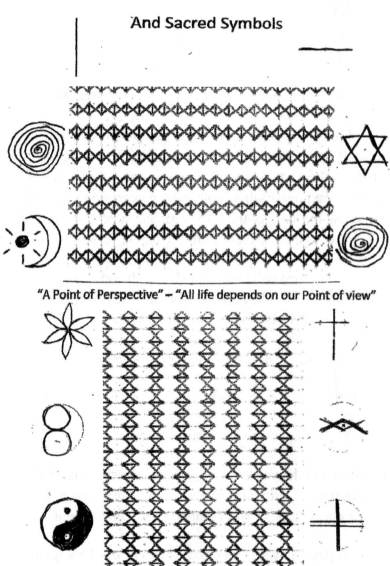

"A Point of Perspective" -- "All life depends on our Point of view"

The universal holographic matrix, and sacred symbols.

A point of perspective. All life depends on our point of view.

We begin to realize our actual ongoing participative, creative role. We are the universal holographic matrix, the holographic reality, creating and experiencing simultaneously.
There was an old cartoon called "Pogo," and one of the characters used to say, "We have met the enemy, and the enemy is us." To paraphrase Pogo, (in a world of peace), "We have met the universal holographic matrix, and the matrix is us."
The adventure begins!

CHAPTER 11

The SHINE Charts

We will access our holographic body and the universal
holographic database using the SHINE charts.

Schley Holographic Information Natural Energy

SHINE = Schley Holographic Information Natural Energy.

You will find the SHINE charts on the following pages. These
charts are a collection of my original graphics and information.
The SHINE chart information is directly related to the title
and subject of the chart. Each SHINE chart has a vast array
of applications (only limited by your imagination) that will
give you access to the holographic body and the universal
holographic database. Combined, with some suggestions for
how to use the SHINE charts, scanning, and muscle testing
can assist you in answering any question you have. We have a
consistent system and charts that we can use for direct physical
experience and discovery. You may even develop your own
methods specific to the nature of your inquiry. This system
is always with us and available, as indicated in chapter 9.
The SHINE charts connect with the cycles and energies of our
body and our universe, when we learn how to read and apply

them. Our bodies are holographic, and our holographic bodies function inside of and as a part of a universal holographic database where all information can be accessed. We are the universal holographic matrix! We are the holographic reality, creating and experiencing simultaneously. Many people, myself included, recognized early on that muscle testing as a biological indicator and information-gathering system had the potential for a much wider application than its conventional uses at the time.

I personally used and still use muscle testing in considerably expanded applications in my practice, including as an indicator of the human body's response to color, and as a tracking tool to identify sources of trauma related to the individual, going back into their history. By 1982, I was using muscle testing for an endless array of applications to access information relating to the body, mind, and spirit. Many other people were researching their areas of interest, using this amazing muscular biofeedback tool. Fast-forward to the present, and we no longer have to prove muscle testing as tool, as there have been millions of credible tests proving muscle testing, and millions of in field applications.

How to Use the SHINE Charts

We can use the SHINE chart, holographic body mandala / holographic body grid, and the holographic body grid (with color vector indicators) to chart the front body and back body energy blocks in the following ways. In chapter 9, we gave a complete example of the process of scanning. The first step is to define what you are looking for or want. The next step is to state your intention and how that intention will occur. If you are using this method for yourself, you may proceed; if you are scanning someone else, you will want to explain the process and intention of that scanning with that person, and get their agreement before proceeding. Here is one method I use. I draw a stick figure on a blank piece of paper and use a pencil to mark the energy blocks on the figure, or I photocopy the appropriate chart/s and mark the energy blocks and related information I need on the chart/s photocopy. (Please do not modify or change the chart's information in any way except to put your scanning information on it, and of course you may take full credit for your specific information, which you should always identify as coming from you and preferably with a date and time.) I state my intention and how it will occur (shown in bold type). The chart I am viewing is my body, or another person's (name, with their permission). I prefer to use a pencil for writing and to scan the body on the chart/s, as the carbon structure of the pencil has a strong harmonic relationship to the holographic body. As I move gently and slowly over the body, my pencil stops at the center (or edge) of any energy block in the body I am scanning. For this, you have to be consciously present to the body you are scanning. If you begin by practicing on your own body, a client, or someone willing to work with you, you can check on your practice by checking those areas on yourself or the person you are working with. I mark each blocked spot and proceed with scanning the rest of the body on the chart/s, marking other areas where the pencil stops until I am complete with the chart/s. If you do not have a chart with you, a stick figure that you draw allows for a quick check, which is always available if you have a blank paper and something to write with. For more detailed charting, you may use the holographic body mandala / holographic body grid chart. You can see that the top half of this chart shows the front body image with two hands and two feet. The two hands are the inside or palm side of the hands, and the two feet are the underside or (inside) of the feet. The bottom half of this chart shows the back of the body, which goes with the outside or fingernail side of the hands, and the outside or toenail side of the feet. This chart allows you to scan and record the energy blocks and their locations on the front and back of the body you are scanning, including the inside and outside of the hands and feet. You may also use the holographic body grid (with color vector indicators) front body and back body.

Scan these charts using the same system described. Scanning first for major blocks and then for minor blocks on the front and back of the body, you will then have a base of information. Now take a deep breath, imagine that breath going to a blocked area, and as you exhale, allow the area to release and balance. You can balance yourself and/or have the person you are working with do the same to balance themselves. If you wish to work with color balancing, you can also use the colors on the chart with the muscle testing instructions that are in chapter 9. The muscle testing instructions are just before the scanning instructions. This will help guide you in beginning to familiarize yourself with color and balancing the body. By learning and using these accurate and valuable systems alone, you will have enough for a lifetime, and you will know that anyone can be introduced to and learn SHINE charts and holographic database and body grid access methods. This and a bit of imagination can expand your universe.

List of SHINE Charts (In Order)

Schley Skin Brushing System
Point and Field Chart
Biosymmetry Chart
Peace Centering Exercise
Color and Balance—Color Field Chart
Color and Balance—Major Energy Vortexes
Universal Holographic Database
Holographic Body Mandala / Holographic Body Grid
Holographic Body Grid (With Color Vector
Indicators, Front and Back Body)
Holographic Body Grid Yin Yang Energy
Flow Charts (Front and Back Body)
Universal Holographic Database and Body Grid Charts
(Two Charts)

Schley Skin Brushing

These two charts consist of a front body and a back body image and instructions for doing the Schley Skin Brushing System (chapter 8 describes this skin brushing system).

Schley Skin Brushing System Chart

1.   Schley Skin Brushing System   4.

SKIN	**BRUSH FROM**
BRUSH	**TOES TO**
FRONT	**HEELS ON**
BODY	**BOTTOM**
FROM	**OF FEET,**
CHEST	**UP**
DOWN	**INSIDE**
INSIDE	**FRONT**
ARMS TO	**OF LEGS,**
HANDS AND	**TORSO, AND**
OUT FINGERS	**CHEST**

Schley Skin Brushing System

Front Body

Schley Skin Brushing System Chart

3.   **Schley Skin Brushing System**   **2.**

FROM TOP   **BRUSH**

OF HEAD   Schley Skin Brushing System   **FINGERS**

DOWN NECK,   **UP BACK**

SHOULDERS   **OF HANDS**

TORSO AND   **ARMS**

LOWER BACK   **OVER**

BUTTOCKS   **SHOULDERS**

THIGHS, LEGS   **AND NECK**

OUTSIDE CALVES   **FACE**

OVER TOP OF   **AND**

FEET AND   **TOP**

OUT TOES   **OF HEAD**

Back Body

Point and Field Chart
Intention and Focus in a Field (Context of Creation)

Point and Field Chart

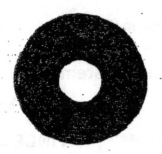

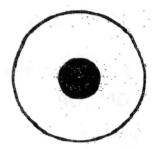

POINT-Where we are at.
We need to be centered to know.

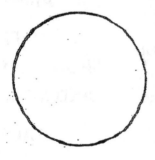

FIELD-Extent of our ability to perceive,
vision, extension of consciousness.

Biosymmetry Chart
(Vector Indicators)

This chart is a photo print of a nested series of closely packed marbles in groups of seven. Relating this chart to the other SHINE charts will help one understand the context of the holographic body as a symmetrical physical grid, without scale or boundary, expanding or contracting energetically and structurally. Whether in a dance of interwoven photons particle/frequencies (light), a structural composite of frozen water molecules (a snowflake), or cells (a living being), the relationship of us to everything is only a matter of focus in a field, aligning itself as a holographic grid.

Biosymmetry Chart

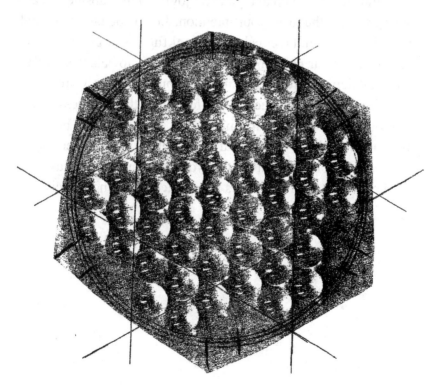

Peace Centering Exercise

Sit comfortably in a chair with your back straight and place both feet on the floor. Imagine that you and your chair are in the center of a sphere, inside a disk or boat. Imagine this disk or boat is a space capsule that you and your chair are comfortably seated inside. This capsule seems to be silver and gold, but when you look out of the capsule, it is totally transparent, and you can see forever in all directions. Breathe gently and deeply and imagine your breath is drawing a circle around you. The in-breath is drawing one side of the circle, and the out-breath is drawing the other side. Think of something in your life that you are thankful for, something that gives you a feeling of thankfulness and gratitude. Imagine as you are sitting there that this feeling of thankfulness and gratitude fills you and you feel joyful. This capsule has a piloting system that uses your intention. Just by being intentional and holding in mind the feeling of thankfulness or gratefulness, we can adjust our body rhythms from chaotic to balance. There is no difficulty here, and all information flows freely around and through you. Appreciate this feeling of thankfulness and gratitude for twenty-four minutes and gently begin to bring your attention back to your starting point. Slowly reenter your present location. You realize that you feel wonderful, relaxed, and peaceful. This completes your peace centering exercise.

Peace Centering Exercise

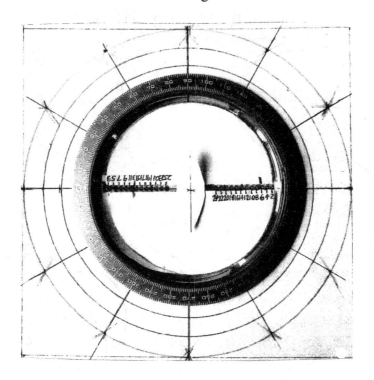

Color and Balance—Color Field Chart

This array represents our holographic body grid.
The grid is a field, and the field is a grid.
Their colors may also be used as points of focus. What
feelings do you have in relation to these colors?
On a separate page, write the name of each color. Write
one dominant feeling you have in relation to each color.

Color and Balance—Color Field Chart

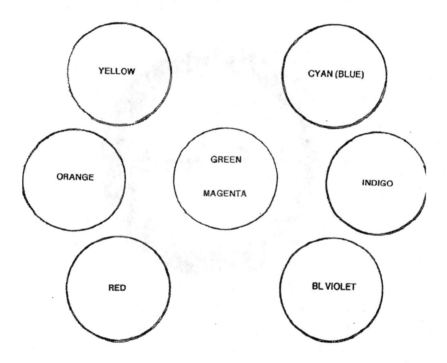

Color and Balance—Major Energy Vortexes
Related to the holographic body grid, this chart
represents seven fields (circles, wheels, or chakras),
each with a specific point of color focus.

Color and Balance—Major Energy Vortexes

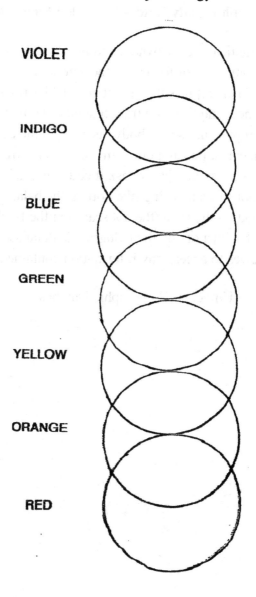

VIOLET

INDIGO

BLUE

GREEN

YELLOW

ORANGE

RED

Universal Holographic Database
Holographic Body Grid—Extended Field Chart

We are energetically everywhere and present. Our reality is a function of our point of focus and the extent of our conscious field. This chart represents a point and field array in which scale, distance, and time are transcended or coincident. This chart could represent us (our body) as a dot in the center circle standing on earth, the first circle in the universe (represented initially as a series of eight circles). It could as easily represent our consciousness focusing (the dot) on the balance of our physical body—the field (the dot scanning the field). Since we are both a part of and the holographic database, we can train ourselves to access any information contained therein.

Universal Holographic Database

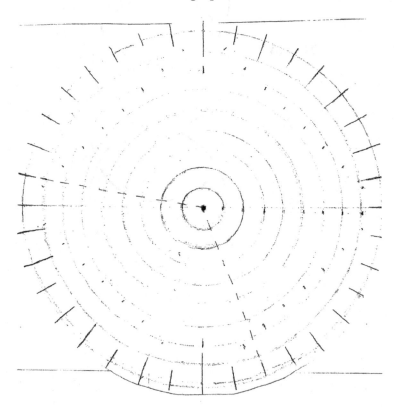

Holographic Body Mandala / Holographic Body Grid Chart

This chart shows the reflex relationship of the hands and feet to the body, and the body relationship to the universal holographic database and the holographic body grid.

Holographic Body Mandala / Holographic Body Grid Chart

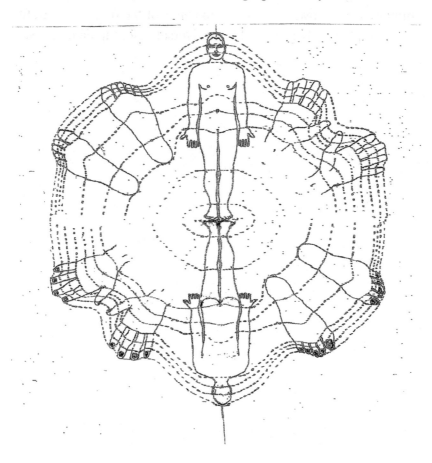

Holographic Body Grid Charts
(With Color Vector Indicators)

These charts, front body, and back body, show an energy pattern
of the universal holographic database as a complementary color-
balanced spectral energy graphic. This flower of life pattern
is portrayed on the physical body in relation to the major and
minor energy flows, vortex relationships of the body to itself, the
holographic body grid, and the universal holographic database.

Front Body

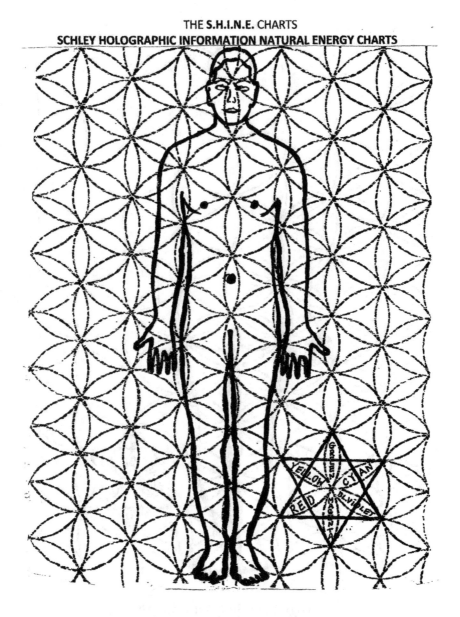

THE **S.H.I.N.E.** CHARTS
SCHLEY HOLOGRAPHIC INFORMATION NATURAL ENERGY CHARTS

Holographic Body Grid Charts
(with color vector indicators)

Back Body

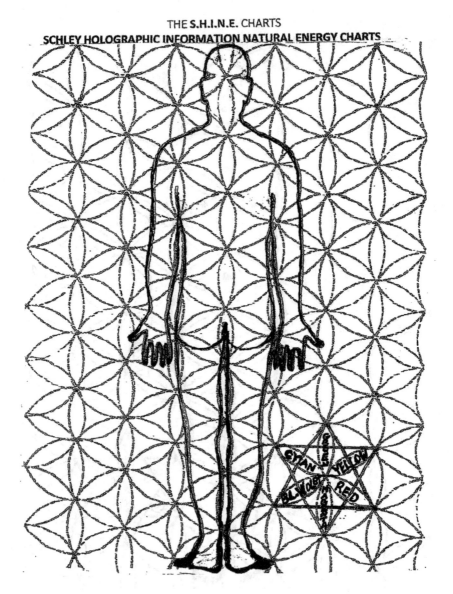

Holographic Body Grid Charts
(with color vector indicators)

Holographic Body Grid Yin Yang Energy Flow Charts

These charts show yin and yang energy
flows on the front and back body.

Front Body

Holographic Body Grid Yin Yang Energy Flow Charts

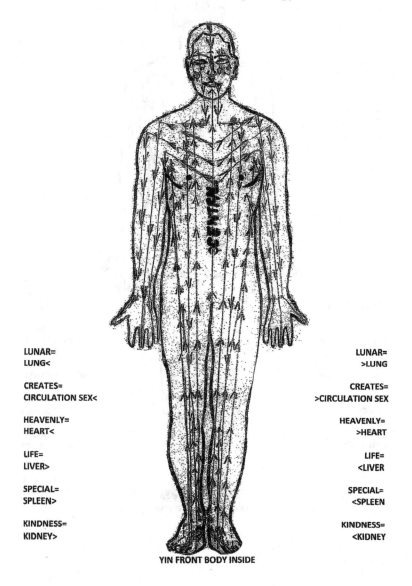

LUNAR=
LUNG<

CREATES=
CIRCULATION SEX<

HEAVENLY=
HEART<

LIFE=
LIVER>

SPECIAL=
SPLEEN>

KINDNESS=
KIDNEY>

LUNAR=
>LUNG

CREATES=
>CIRCULATION SEX

HEAVENLY=
>HEART

LIFE=
<LIVER

SPECIAL=
<SPLEEN

KINDNESS=
<KIDNEY

YIN FRONT BODY INSIDE

Back Body

Holographic Body Grid Yin Yang Energy Flow Charts

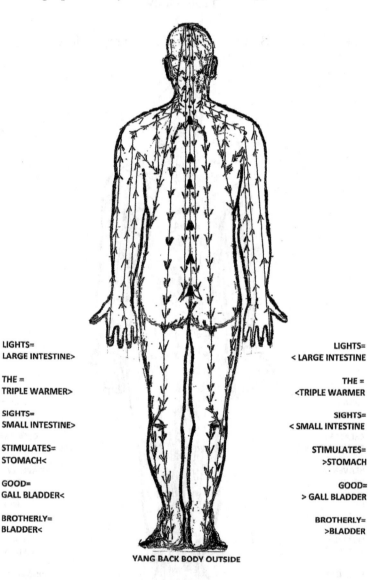

LIGHTS= LARGE INTESTINE>	LIGHTS= < LARGE INTESTINE
THE = TRIPLE WARMER>	THE = <TRIPLE WARMER
SIGHTS= SMALL INTESTINE>	SIGHTS= < SMALL INTESTINE
STIMULATES= STOMACH<	STIMULATES= >STOMACH
GOOD= GALL BLADDER<	GOOD= > GALL BLADDER
BROTHERLY= BLADDER<	BROTHERLY= >BLADDER

YANG BACK BODY OUTSIDE

Schley Holographic Information Natural Energy Charts
Universal Holographic Database and Body Grid

These two charts show how all the other charts relate and
synchronize with each other, regardless of scale, time,
or distance in an ongoing celebration of the present.

Universal Holographic Database and Body Grid

These two charts show a twelve-by-twelve grid overlaid on a
circle. The first chart is the twelve-by-twelve grid overlaid on a
polar array divided into thirty-degree segments with different
sizes of circles, squares, and lines that could be an endless series
of different things, but no matter what the size, shape, or location,
they show a similar relationship to each other. The grid could,
for example, represent a universe section of twelve-by-twelve
light years square with navigational coordinates, or the seven
major chakras of our body on a twenty-four-hour grid. What
it is showing is the yin/yang movement of energy through the
twelve major bilateral meridians of our body and the exact time
and directional energy relationship to a twenty-four-hour, noon
to midnight back to noon, time period. It also does show the
seven major chakras of the body on a twenty-four-hour grid.
In addition, if we look closely, we can see the two fish and five
loaves of bread (holographic array strand) mentioned earlier in this
book. The fish tails are visible at the top and bottom of the center
section of stacked circles (chakras). Once you see the fish, it will
be easy to see the five diamond-shape loaves between the two fish
$(2 + 5 = 7$, the major chakras array of our body). This represents
one partial strand of an endless array of strands, both macro and
micro of our infinitely connected holographic body and universe.
The second chart shows the same twelve-by-twelve grid
as a universal number array (all reference points have two
numbers, and all add up to twelve). This is a graphic indicator

of a holographic grid where each point contains the whole. Looking carefully, we will also see patterns of odd and even number sequences that repeat symmetrically throughout the system. This array contains all possibilities of structure, scale, and dimension. All secrets of life and form are hidden in and can be modeled using this array. It is holographic! Using just the information on these charts and muscle testing, we can tell what direction of energy movement will strengthen the body and help someone balance their chakra system. Using muscle testing and the yin/yang energy flow charts in this chapter, you can tell what energy meridians are out of balance. Often just doing the Schley Skin Brushing System will balance the meridians. On the yin/yang energy flow charts, once you have discovered using muscle testing what meridians are out of balance, you can often balance the body by reflex massage along the energy flow lines, following the direction of flow indicated by the arrows, or the flow as described in the Skin Brushing System. There is an infinite number of ways presented in this book for you to achieve, or to coach someone else to achieve a more balanced and healthy body. Just doing what is suggested in this book will guarantee it.

The adventure begins!

SCHLEY HOLOGRAPHIC INFORMATION NATURAL ENERGY CHARTS
UNIVERSAL HOLOGRAPHIC DATABASE AND BODY GRID

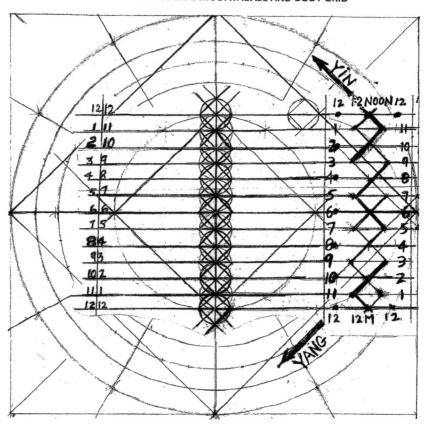

SCHLEY HOLOGRAPHIC INFORMATION NATURAL ENERGY CHARTS
UNIVERSAL HOLOGRAPHIC DATABASE AND BODY GRID

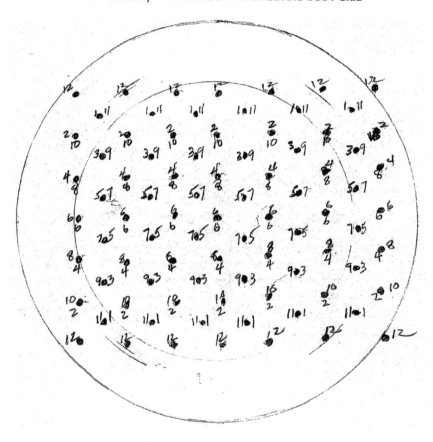

CHAPTER 12

Peace—A Simple State of Being

Peace is defined as a normal state of mutual harmony between people or groups getting along with each other. The entire physical universe is always seeking balance; acids seek alkaline, alkaline seeks acid, hot cools, cool warms. On earth, high water and low water seek to be even water. Whether you raise or lower a transparent tube filled with water, it stays even.

Water-------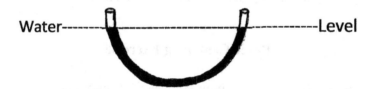------Level

Our physical body is also continually seeking to be balanced; this is called seeking homeostasis, also called a state of balance. The state of balance has another word, and this word is peace. We can say we live in an apparently chaotic three-dimensional world that is always seeking peace. The good news is that peace is always present! The question is, are we experiencing peace? Are we experiencing peace at all levels of our physical, mental, emotional, and spiritual existence? When we are experiencing peace in these areas, everything occurs as what we call good. We have good health, good thoughts, good emotions, good spirit. This experience, or state of being, we call peace or balance. The good news is we get to choose. The bad news we often do not get the presents in our life, recognizing we get to choose. We often experience life as "that's just the way it is right now." Choice is always present if we are aware of it. How do we choose peace? What do we do next? Honor our friends and allow space for everyone to be our friend. Connect at the heart, recognize our oneness, and peace is present. Say, "I commit to being a peaceful person. I practice being a peaceful person. I experience being a peaceful person. I mentor being a peaceful person. I am peace. I practice peace. I share peace." When we "live" backwards, we have "evil." Love must be present to evolve! "We need more picnics," said His Holiness the Dali Lama. Make friends, and have your friends make friends. Tell wonderful stories. The best stories win the present. Once upon a time, there were and still are people you love, and who love you, and don't forget: KISSES= Keep It Simple Sweetheart Ever Simple!

Please do the peace centering exercise from Chapter 11. SHINE charts now. Thank you

Peace Centering Exercise

Sit comfortably in a chair with your back straight and place both feet flat on the floor. Imagine that you and your chair are in the center of a sphere, inside a disk or boat. Imagine this disk or boat is a space capsule that you and your chair are comfortably seated inside. This capsule seems to be silver and gold, but when you look out of the capsule, it is totally transparent, and you can see forever in all directions. Breathe gently and deeply and imagine your breath is drawing a circle around you. The in-breath is drawing one side of the circle, and the out-breath is drawing the other side. Think of something in your life that you are thankful for, something that gives you a feeling of thankfulness and gratitude. Imagine as you are sitting there that this feeling of thankfulness and gratitude fills you, and you feel joyful. This capsule has a piloting system that uses your intention. Just by being intentional and holding in mind the feeling of thankfulness or gratefulness, we can adjust our body rhythms from chaotic to balance. There is no difficulty here, and all information and energy flows freely around and through you. Appreciate this feeling of thankfulness and gratitude for twenty-four minutes and gently begin to bring your attention back to your starting point. Slowly reenter your present location. You realize that you feel wonderful, relaxed, and peaceful. This completes your peace centering exercise.

CHAPTER 13

Are We Having Fun? Being Grateful, Thankful, Allowing—Now. It's All Energy and the Point.

You are now at the thirteenth chapter of a thirteen-chapter book, and hopefully you have discovered some of the hidden treasures and are already experiencing your own adventure— or have realized you were living it all along. Or perhaps you realized that you were not having fun, and you have chosen to make a change, and that change is in progress. If you have been paying attention, you have learned how to answer any question you may have in life, and you have started answering your life questions and adjusting your life so that it better serves you and others. Thank you for reading this book! Even the words *thank you* are whole (holy). I believe (thank you) T ANKH U was derived from a ceremonial act of healing—a whole (holy) person sharing at the heart level with another. Imagine a person laying on a table face up with their feet together and their arms outstretched, another person at their head with both of their arms extended, touching the person on the table with one hand over the other, at the heart level. T ANKH U. Looking from above, this would be a physical representation of sharing at the heart level. This heart sharing may have been represented in the form of what we have come to know as the Egyptian ankh, used as a symbol of healing, enduring life, sharing, or regeneration.

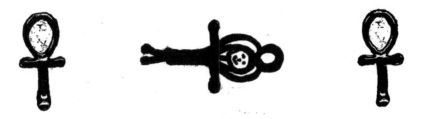

Thankful, Allowing, Being—Now

Being thankful is to heal. Allowing is to get out of the way. Allow yourself to receive the present. Being is now. It's all energy. We live in an apparently three-dimensional world, yet there is far more space than matter and many more dimensions than we are consciously aware of. We have access to all of life, all information, all possibility. There is nothing in our way. When we choose to be determines where we are. Keep this book and apply it; it is a treasure. Read it again and again. Each time you will find something new—and the point. Now the adventure begins.

BIBLIOGRAPHY

(References and Resources by Chapter)

1. Breathing

Beck, Melinda. "What Your Breath Reveals." *Wall Street Journal.*
Dinshah Ghadiali Dinshah. S*pectrochrometry Encyclopedia,* vols. 1–3. (New Jersey: Health Society).
Fletcher, Edna Adelia. *The Law of Rhythmic Breathing.*
Iyengar B.K.S. *Yoga (The Path to Holistic Health).*
Jwing Ming, Dr. Yang. *The Root of Chinese Qigong (Secrets for Health, Longevity, and Enlightenment).*
Russel, Walter. *The Secret of Light.* 233.
Yee, Rodney. *Yoga the Poetry of the Body.*

2. Water

Bragg, Paul. *Water, The Shocking Truth That Can Save Your Life.*
Emoto, Masaru. *Hidden Messages in Water.* 2004.
Page, Linda Rector, N.D., Ph.D. *Healthy Healing.*
Salzman, Michael H. *New Water for a Thirsty World.* 1960.

3. Food

Bittman, Mark. *How to Cook Everything (Simple Recipes for Great Food).*
Davidson, Alan. *The Oxford Companion to Food.*
Doutre-Roussel, Chloe. *The Chocolate Connoisseur, For Everyone with a Passion for Chocolate.*

Engleheart, Terces with Orchid. *I Am Grateful (Recipes and Lifestyle of Café Gratitude).*

Horn, Jane (editor/writer) and Janet Fletcher (contributing writer) *Cooking A to Z.*

Jensen, Dr. Bernard. *Dr. Jensen's Guide to Body Chemistry and Nutrition.* Jensen, Dr. Bernard. *Foods That Heal.*

Lebovitz, David. *My Paris Kitchen.*

Lebovitz, David. *The Great Book of Chocolate.*

Mueller, Tom. *Extra Virginity—The Sublime and Scandalous World of Olive Oil.*

Nabhan, Paul. *Where Our Food Comes From (Retracing Nicolay Vasilov's Quest to End Famine).*

Pfeiffer, Ehrenfried and Michael Maltas. *The Biodynamic Orchard Book.*

Pfeiffer, Ehrenfried. *Pfeiffer's Introduction to Biodynamics.*

Robbins, John. *The Food Revolution (How your Diet Can Save Your Life and Our World).*

Roberts, Wayne. *The No-Nonsense Guide to World Food.*

Rosenblum, Mort. *Chocolate (A Bittersweet Saga of Dark and Light).*

Rosenblum, Mort. *Olives (The Life and Lore of a Noble Fruit).*

Sanmi, Sasaki. *Chado—The Way of Tea (A Japanese Tea Master's Almanac),* translated from the Japanese by Shaun McCabe and Iwasaki Satoko, foreword by Sen Soshitsu XV, grand tea master of the Urasenke School.

Schley, Vicki Barrios and Angelo Villa. *Mexican Cooking at the Academy (California Culinary Academy).* Susan Lammers, ed.

Shurtleff, William and Akiko Aoyagi. *The Book of Miso (Food for Mankind).*

Patel, Raj. *Stuffed and Starved (The Hidden Battle for the World Food System).*

The Whole Seed Catalog. (Baker Creek Heirloom Seeds).

Ukers, William H. *All About Coffee.*

Weissman, Michaele. *God in a Cup (The Obsessive Quest for the Perfect Cup (of Coffee).*

Wolfe, David and Shazzie. *Naked Chocolate—The Astonishing Truth about the World's Greatest Food.*
Wright, Hilary. *Biodynamic Gardening for Health and Taste.*

4. Herbivore, Omnivore, Carnivore

Pollan, Michael. *In Defense of Food: An Eater's Manifesto.*
Pollan, Michael. *The Omnivore's Dilemma.*

5. Exercise

Ellsworth, Dr. Abigail. *Anatomy of Yoga.*
Iyengar, B.K.S. *Yoga (The Path to Holistic Health).*
Yee, Rodney. *Yoga the Poetry of the Body.*

6. Simplify, Adjust Your Use and Consumption

Pierce, Linda Breen. Choosing Simplicity (Real people finding peace and fulfilment in a complex world)
Clark, Corie. The Simplicity Project: (Win your battle with chaos and clutter so you can live a life of peace and purpose).
Hanh, Thich Nhat. Being Peace.

7. Environmental Living

Mother Earth Living.
Mother Earth News.

8. Body Cleansing, the Schley Skin Brushing System, and Fasting

Ehret, Professor Arnold. *Rational Fasting.*

9. Health, Color, and Healing

Brennan, Barbara Ann. *Hands of Light.*
Ghadiali, Dinshah. Spectrochrometry Encyclopedia, vols. 1–3. New Jersey: Health Society.
Gawain, Shakti. *Living in the Light.*
Hawkins, David R., MD, PhD. *Power Vs Force (The Hidden Determinants of Human Behavior).*

Hay, Louise. *You Can Heal Your Life*.

Krieger, Dolores. *The Therapeutic Touch*.

Kuppers, Harald. *Color, Origin, System, Uses*.

Liberman, Jacob. *Light: Medicine of the Future*.

Page. Linda Rector, N.D., Ph.D. Healthy Healing.

Targ, Russell and Harold Puthoff. *Mind*.

New York: Delacorte Press, 1973.

Thie, Dr. John. *Touch for Health*.

Weintraub, Skye, ND. *Natural Healing with Cell Salts*.

10. Holographic Body Transcends the Imagining—Or Does It?

Blechschmidt, Erich. *The Ontogenetic Basis of Human Anatomy, a Biodynamic Approach to Development from Conception to Birth*, edited and translated by Brian Freeman.

Bohm, David. *Hidden Variables and the Implicate Order*.

Golas, Thaddeus. *The Lazy Man's Guide to Enlightenment*.

Hanh, Thich Nhat. Living Buddha, Living Christ, and tenth anniversary edition.

Hills, Christopher. *Nuclear Evolution*.

Hills, Christopher. *Supersensonics*.

His Holiness the Dalai Lama. *The Universe in a Single Atom, The Convergence of Science and Spirituality*.

Holy Bible Revised Standard Version, Old and New Testaments, Translated from the original tongues being the version set forth AD 1611, revised AD 1881–1885 and AD 1901, compared with the most ancient authorities and revised AD 1952, Thomas Nelson & Sons.

Judith, Anodea, PhD. *The Global Heart Awakens, Humanity's Rite of Passage from the Love of Power to the Power of Love*.

Kushi, Michio. *Oriental Diagnosis, What Your Face Reveals*.

Melchizedek, Drunvalo. *The Ancient Secret of the Flower of Life*, volume 1 and volume 2.

Myss, Caroline, PhD. *Anatomy of the Spirit, the Seven Stages of Power and Healing*.

Schley, Michael A. *Master Series: Secret of Everything, Your Adventure Begins*.

Talbot, Michael. *The Holographic Universe.*
Van Beek, Wil. *Hazrat Inayat Khan.* New York: Vantage Press.
Wilbur, Ken and Carlo McCormick. *Sacred
Mirrors, The Visionary Art of Alex Grey.*
Yogananda, Paramhansa. *Autobiography of a Yogi.*
Los Angeles: Self-Realization Fellowship, 1973.
Zukav, Gary. *The Seat of the Soul.*

11. The SHINE Charts

12. Peace—A Simple State of Being

Childre, Doc Lew. *The HeartMath Solution.*

13. Are We Having Fun? Grateful, Thankful, Allowing, Being—Now. It's All Energy and the Point.

The Ankh Key of Life by the editors of Weiser
Books, introduction by Lon Milo Duquette.

ABOUT THE AUTHOR

Michael leads health, peace, color, bodywork, and universal holographic database access workshops. He is a public speaker, plays guitar, is an artist, writes poems and songs, and continues his successful now 37th year health consulting, life coaching, and holographic bodywork practice.

Printed in the United States
By Bookmasters

Printed in the United States
By Bookmasters